5-MINUTE

—— WORKOUTS FOR SENIORS ——

STRENGTH TRAINING

Your 4-Week Journey to Reclaim Vitality. Low Impact Illustrated Exercises for Robust Bones, Youthful Mobility, and Elevated Stamina

EVELYN TURNER

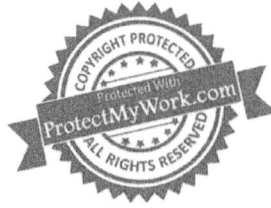

TABLE OF CONTENT

EXERCISES FLOWS

WARM-UP EXERCISES

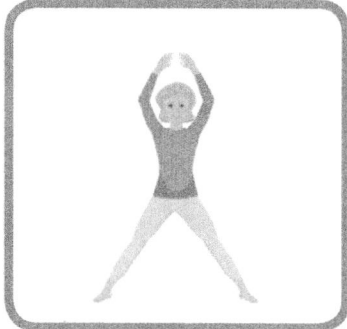

JUMPING JACKS
PAG. 31

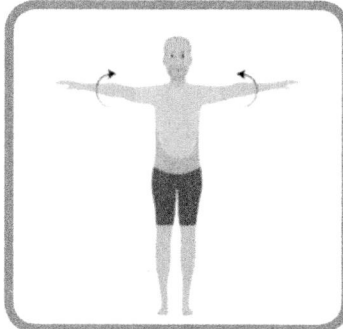

ARM CIRCLES
PAG. 32

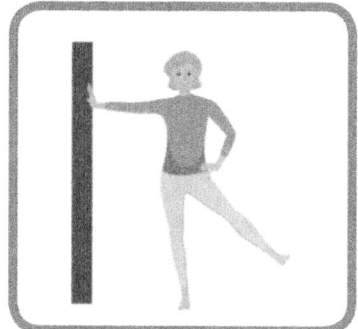

LEG SWINGS
PAG. 33

STRENGTH AND RESISTANCE EXERCISES

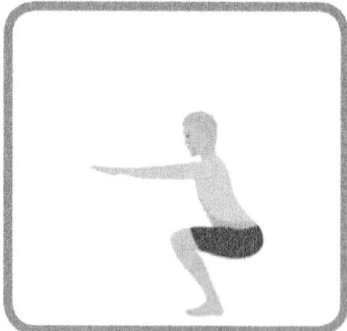

BODYWEIGHT SQUATS
PAG. 34

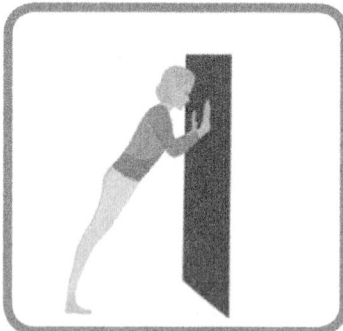

WALL PUSH-UPS
PAG. 35

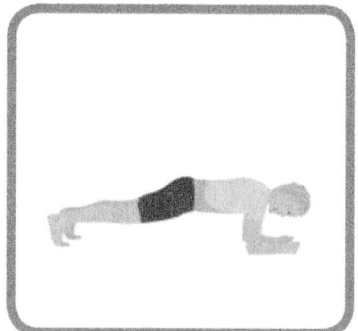

PLANK
PAG. 36

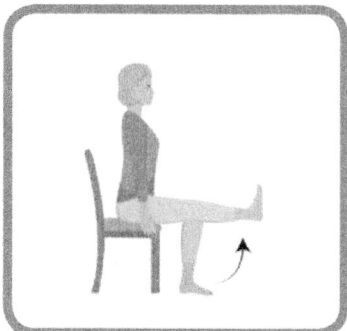

SEATED LEG-RAISES
PAG. 37

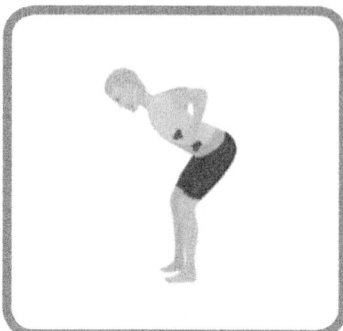

BENT-OVER DUMBBELL ROWS
PAG. 38

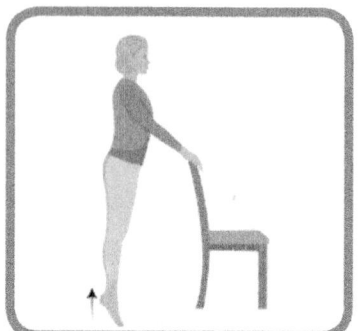

STANDING LEG CALF-RAISES
PAG. 39

STRENGTH AND RESISTANCE EXERCISES

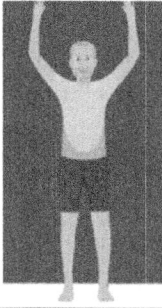

**WALL ANGELS
PAG. 40**

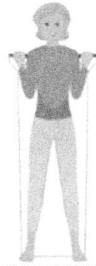

**RESISTANCE BAND BICEP CURL
PAG. 41**

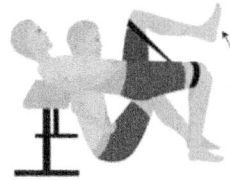

**KNEE EXTENSIONS WITH
RESISTANCE BAND
PAG. 42**

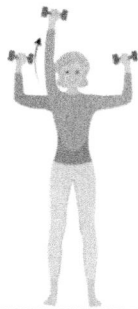

**STANDING DUMBBELL
SHOULDER PRESS
PAG. 43**

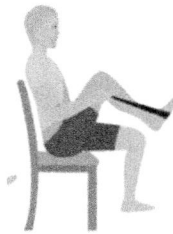

**SEATED LEG PRESS (USING A
RESISTANCE BAND)
PAG. 44**

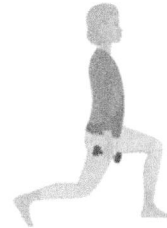

**DUMBBELL LUNGES
PAG. 45**

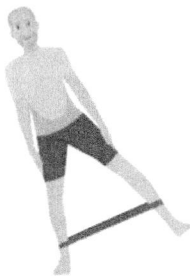

**RESISTANCE BAND LEG
ABDUCTION
PAG. 46**

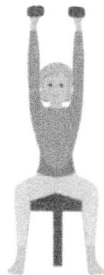

**SEATED DUMBBELL
SHOULDER PRESS
PAG. 47**

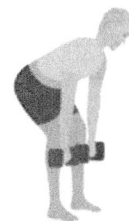

**BENT KNEE DEADLIFTS
PAG. 48**

STRENGTH AND RESISTANCE EXERCISES

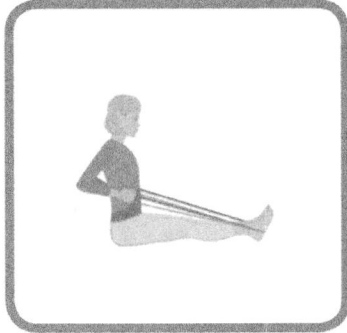

**SEATED ROWS
(MACHINE/RESISTANCE BAND)
PAG. 49**

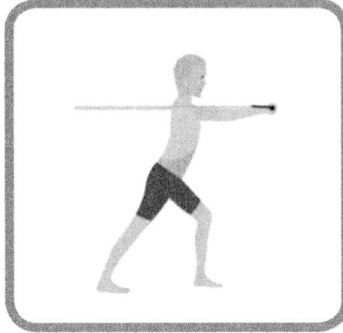

**RESISTANCE BAND
CHEST PRESS
PAG. 50**

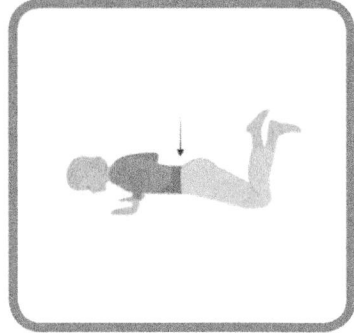

**BENT KNEE PUSH-UPS
PAG. 51**

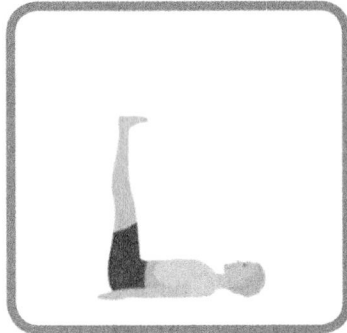

**LYING LEG RAISES
PAG. 52**

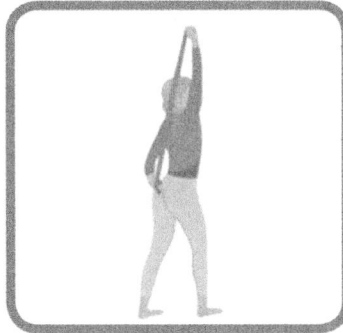

**RESISTANCE BAND
TRICEP STRETCH
PAG. 53**

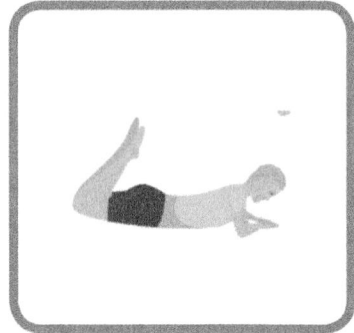

**LYING LEG CURLS
PAG. 54**

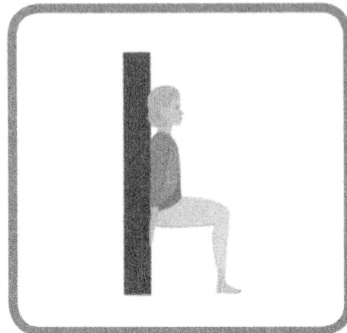

**WALL SIT
PAG. 55**

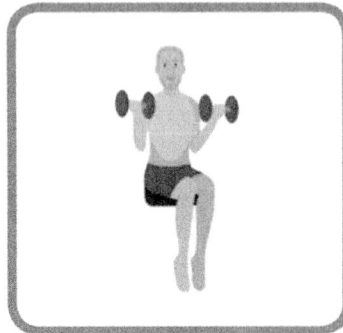

**SEATED BICEP CURL
PAG. 56**

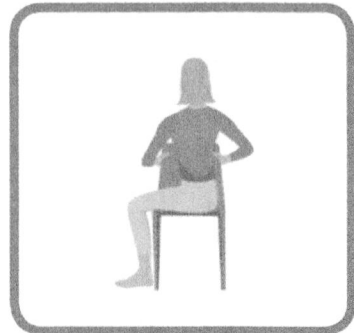

**SIDE TWISTS
PAG. 57**

STRENGTH AND RESISTANCE EXERCISES

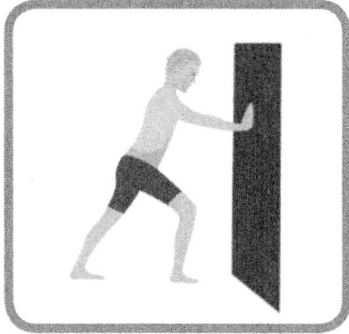

CALF STRETCHES
PAG. 58

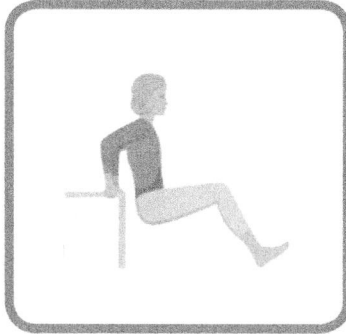

CHAIR DIPS
PAG. 59

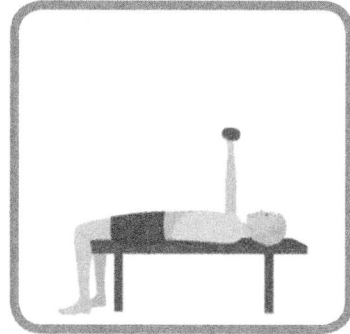

CHEST PRESS
PAG. 60

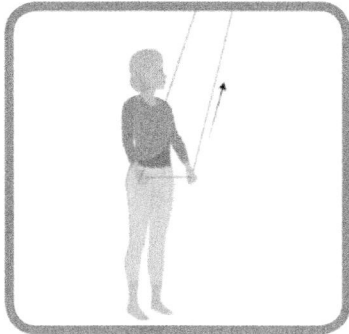

RESISTANCE BAND
LAT PULLDOWNS
PAG. 61

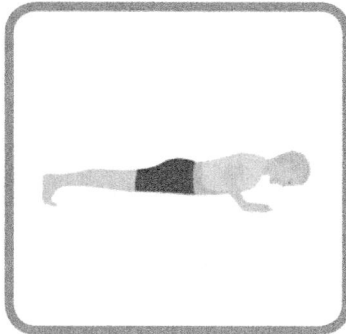

PUSH-UPS
PAG. 62

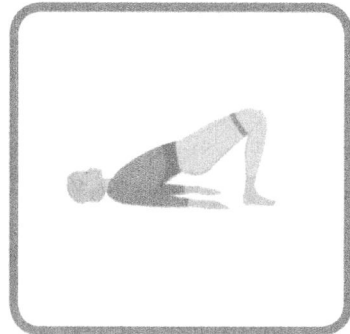

GLUTE BRIDGE
PAG. 63

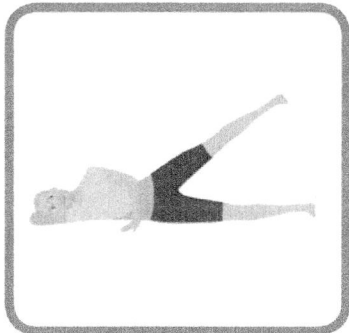

SIDE LEG RAISES
PAG. 64

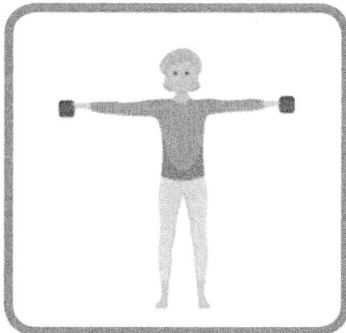

DUMBBELL SIDE RAISES
PAG. 65

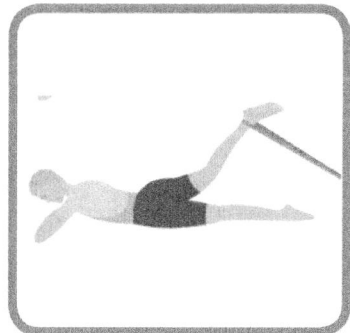

RESISTANCE BAND
LEG CURLS
PAG. 66

STRENGTH AND RESISTANCE EXERCISES

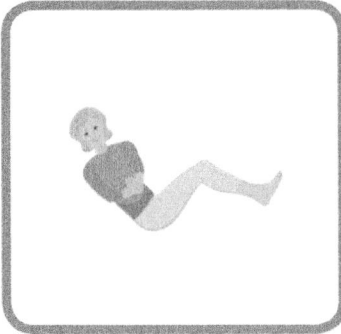

SEATED RUSSIAN TWISTS
PAG. 67

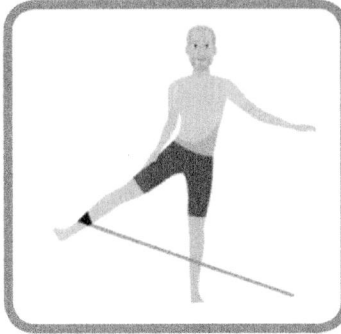

RESISTANCE BAND
HIP ABDUCTION
PAG. 68

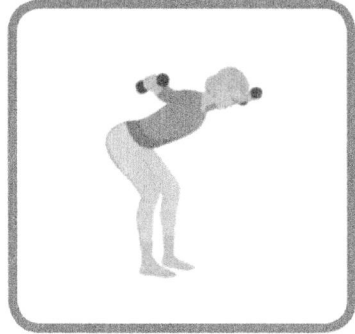

DUMBBELL BENT-OVER
REVERSE FLYES
PAG. 69

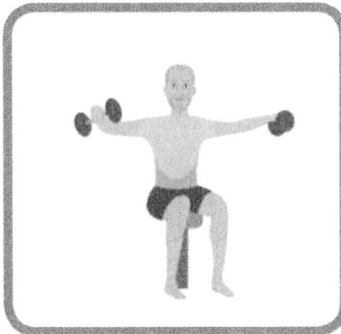

SEATED LATERAL RAISES
PAG. 70

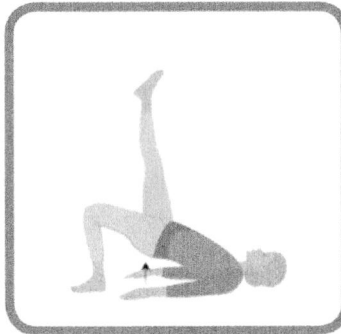

BRIDGE WITH LEG LIFTS
PAG. 71

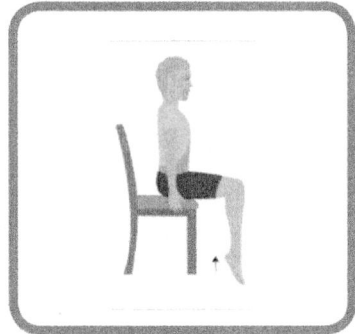

SEATED CALF RAISES
PAG. 72

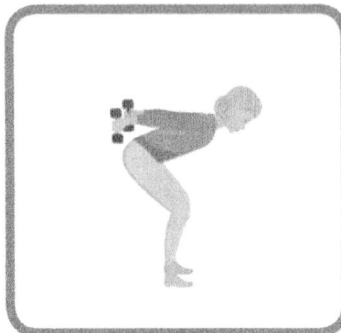

DUMBBELL TRICEP KICKBACKS
PAG. 73

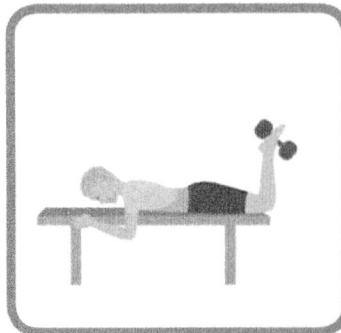

LYING HAMSTRING CURLS
WITH WEIGHTS
PAG. 74

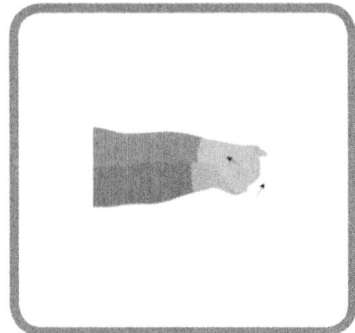

FOREARM STRETCH
PAG. 75

STRENGTH AND RESISTANCE EXERCISES

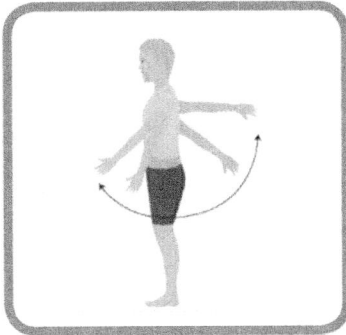

ARM SWINGS
PAG. 76

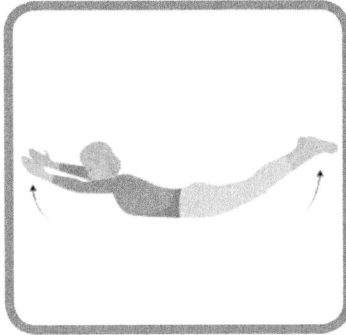

SUPERMAN
PAG. 77

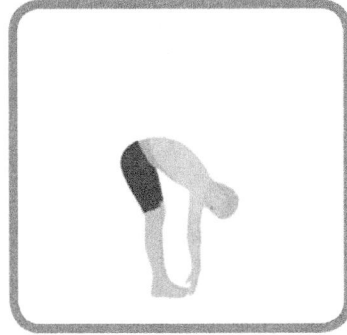

TOE TOUCHES
PAG. 78

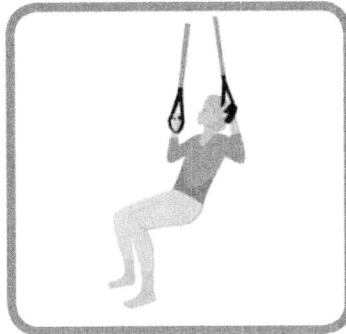

HANGING LAT STRETCH
PAG. 79

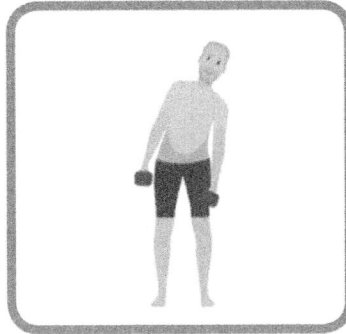

SIDE BENDS
PAG. 80

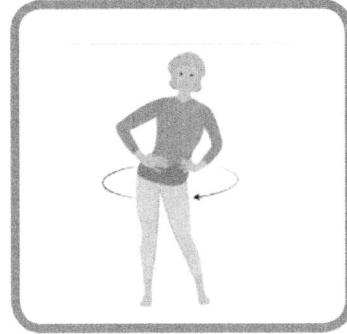

HIP CIRCLES
PAG. 81

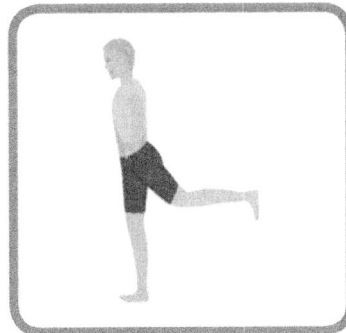

LEG SWINGS
PAG. 82

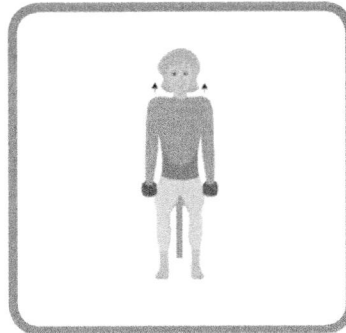

SEATED DUMBBELL SHRUGS
PAG. 83

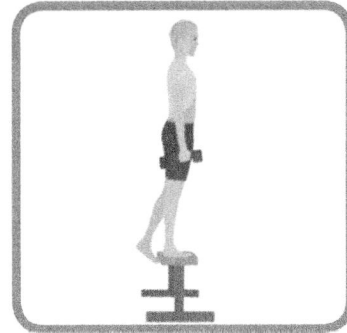

DUMBBELL STEP-UPS
PAG. 84

STRENGTH AND RESISTANCE EXERCISES

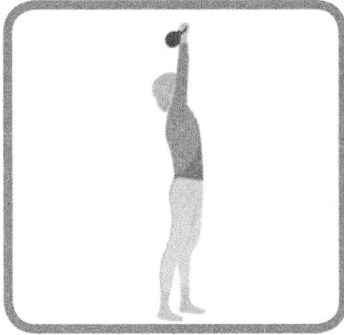

**TURKISH GET-UP
PAG. 85**

COOL DOWN STRETCHES

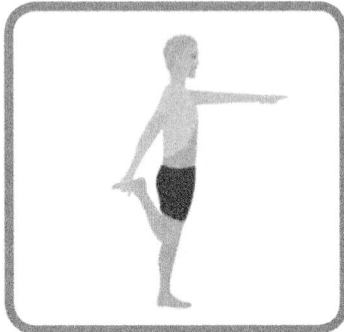

**QUADRICEPS STRETCH
PAG. 86**

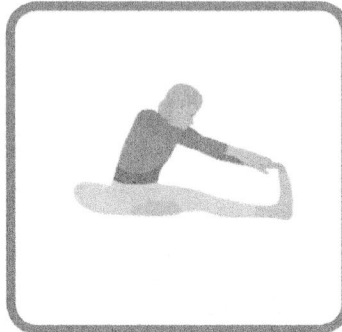

**HAMSTRING STRETCH
PAG. 87**

INTRODUCTION

The world of strength training for seniors is fraught with myths, misinformation, and at times, a lot of excuses about why we cannot become stronger, healthier, and more vibrant in our golden years. And I am not denying I didn't fall into this category myself—that is until I recaptured my zest for life and understood the importance of becoming strong as I aged. This is also why I wrote *5-Minute Strength Training Workouts for Seniors: Your 4-Week Journey to Reclaim Vitality. Low Impact Illustrated Exercises for Robust Bones, Youthful Mobility, and Elevated Stamina*—to demystify strength training for seniors.

I wanted to create a practical book that every senior can use to embark on a journey of shedding stereotypes about strength training and the age-old adage that we become fragile when we enter into our golden years. Now, before I continue with this introduction, and the subsequent chapters, I'd like for us to take a moment to visualize a scene—picture this: a group of friends in their 60s and 70s, laughing together in a local park. They're not there for a leisurely stroll or slowly ambling as their bones and muscles ache and strain. They're in the park to complete a 5-minute strength training routine that has become the highlight of their day. As they lift small weights, stretch their muscles, and support each other through the exercises, each senior shows their strength and determination by completing every rep methodically and with ease.

Now what if I told you this isn't the exception, but the norm—or at least it should be… Strength training is often associated with youth and athleticism, but in reality, it's for everyone and is one of the most beneficial activities seniors can undertake. It's the key that unlocks the door to independence, fall prevention, and enjoying a high quality of life as they get older. And the best part? You don't need to spend hours in the gym to become stronger, fitter, and more capable in your senior year. With just 5 minutes per day, *you* can change your life for the better.

Now, these three seniors aren't random people; they're inspiring friends I have made while teaching *5-Minute Strength Training Workouts for Seniors*.

Jane was 68 years old when I first met her. She had experienced her fair share of life's challenges, battling through health issues, including arthritis and osteoporosis, and found herself feeling increasingly limited in her daily activities. Simple tasks like carrying groceries or climbing stairs were a challenge and Jane knew she needed to make a change.

With the encouragement of her daughter, Jane started her journey to *5-Minute Strength Training,* first at home, then at the community center, and finally with her park-going group of friends. Her journey may seem like a slow one, using light dumbbells and resistance bands to begin with but over time she gradually increased the intensity as she grew stronger. What started as a few minutes of exercise each day soon became a source of pride and accomplishment for Jane and in a few months, Jane was not only moving more easily but also taking up new hobbies like gardening and hiking.

Jane met George, a 72-year-old retired teacher who, at first, couldn't wait to enjoy his retired life to the fullest. However, he quickly realized that his energy levels were dwindling as he fell into the trap of living a more sedentary, less demanding life. With his muscle mass being lost at an alarming rate and frustrated by his loss of vitality, George decided to take action.

Under my guidance at the community center, George started a 5-minute strength training routine that targeted his specific needs. He combined his strength training with regular walks in the park and changed up his nutrition to support his muscle growth. Over time, George not only regained his lost muscle but also discovered he could, in fact, build muscle in his senior years. George now volunteers at his local library and even took up dancing with one of our other seniors. George taught me that it's never too late to reverse the effects of aging and rediscover the things we are passionate about in life.

Finally, Sarah, a 65-year-old grandmother joined our community class after suffering a motor vehicle accident. Since the accident, Sarah had found that she felt older and more fragile. She had experienced a few falls that left her feeling vulnerable and fearful of growing older, but Sarah was determined that she wouldn't lose her independence. Determined to make a change, Sarah embarked on a 5-minute strength training journey that incorporated balance exercises to prevent falls. She found support from friends at the community center and the camaraderie drove her motivation to succeed. Slowly but surely, Sarah's confidence grew and so did her strength and balance. Let me tell you, Sarah not only found her confidence, but she really embraced it and now joins her grandchildren in their outdoor adventures, hiking and biking along with them.

These are just a few examples of the incredible transformations that can happen when seniors embrace the power of strength training. In this book, we will explore the science behind strength training, the benefits it offers, and most importantly, provide a simple and effective 5-minute routine tailored specifically for seniors. You'll learn how to perform each exercise safely and effectively, and we'll debunk the myths and misconceptions that may have held you back.

These three seniors are some of many who have embraced their journey to strength and independence. It doesn't matter if you're in your 60s, 70s, or beyond, it's time to embrace your own journey to strength and vitality. It's going to take dedication and guidance but that's why I am on this journey with you. Now is the time to rewrite your narrative about aging and embrace the idea that you too can become stronger, healthier, and more resilient in your golden years. Let's get started on this transformative journey together.

Today is the first day of *Your 4-Week Journey to Reclaim Vitality. Low Impact Illustrated Exercises for Robust Bones, Youthful Mobility, and Elevated Stamina*–Let's begin.

Chapter 1
STRENGTH IN THE GOLDEN YEARS

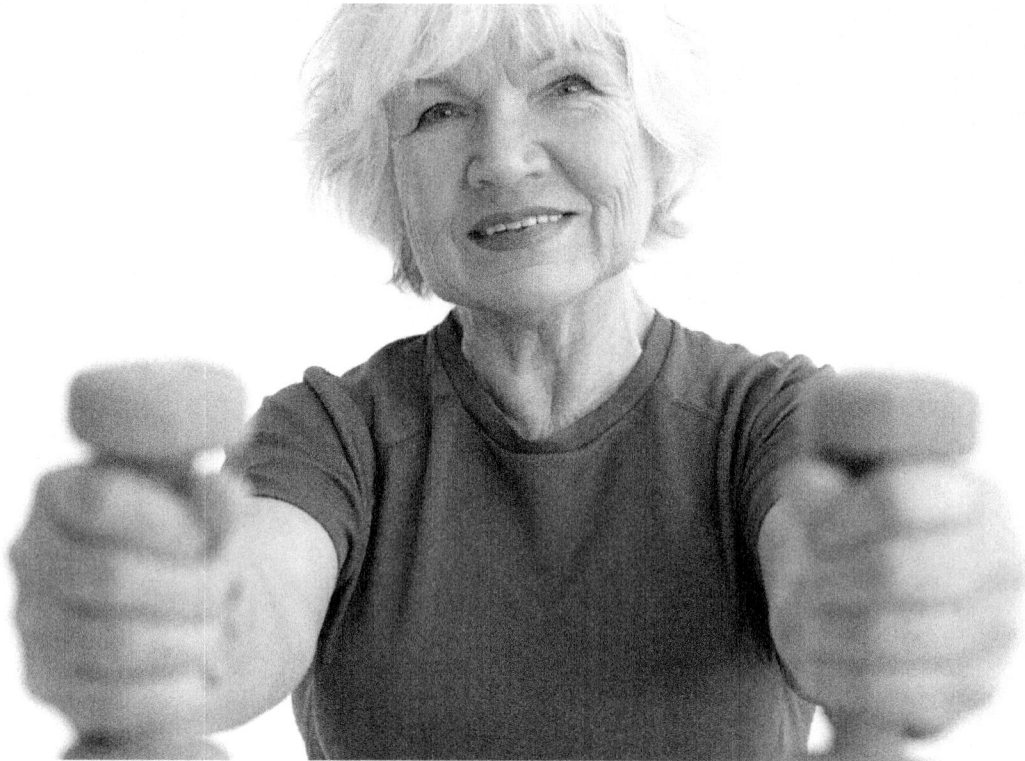

I like to start my classes at the local community center by reminding each of the people that this is our golden years. It's a time when we look back and see how far we have come. We have gone through our teenage and adult years with passion, vigor, and dedication. All of this has led up until now when we have begun showing signs of the aging process. We are looking at ourselves in the mirror, and we see those wrinkles on our skin, the gray in our hair, and the hunch in our back and shoulders.

This does happen to be the natural order of aging. There are no set rules on how you need to behave and live during this time in your life. The most common belief is that after you reach your senior years and you retire from your profession it's time to sit down, relax, and enjoy that sedentary lifestyle. It does sound very inviting and most of us feel that we deserve this. After all, we have been working most of our lives to earn a living and we have made the right decisions, learned from our mistakes, and have come this far, so what's stopping us from taking a break and getting all that rest that we need? The issue with this type of lifestyle is that there are side effects from choosing to let go of what you have worked hard for all this time. You are letting go of something that came naturally during your younger years—your strength. It may seem irrelevant. Why would an older individual need strength? It's not as though you're going to be participating in any strenuous physical activities and you definitely won't need it for a day job. This is unwise and untrue. Throughout my years, I always remained active but during my senior year, I did take some time off thinking that I deserved a little break. After retiring, I wanted to relax and enjoy myself. This was not the best decision. I began to notice that I was putting on weight. My anxiety levels slowly increased as I suddenly felt overwhelmed whenever I did anything like walking or climbing up a few stairs. I imagined I would easily fall and injure myself.

On the other hand, it was becoming increasingly challenging to maintain my physical fitness because of the related limitations of aging. I began to develop mild arthritis, which prevented me from participating in more intense physical activities. I did not want to injure myself during any exercise, which was partly why I chose to just do nothing for a long while. This all led me to become a much lonelier individual. I must go on to add that I do enjoy having an active lifestyle and a positive outlook on life. Things had to change and I could not allow my mind and body to wither away. It was as though I had sentenced myself to a slow deterioration. I did not want this anymore.

My patience and persistence helped prepare me for the new journey where I wanted to change the way I had begun living my senior years. I wanted to be sociable and stay connected with not only my family but my friends as well. The only answer to all of my issues was to go back out there and stay active. My doctor often emphasizes the importance of regular exercise, especially strength training. Eventually, I began to hear stories from my friends about how their health problems were increasing and affecting their lifestyles. They also tried to follow their doctor's advice but had very bad experiences continuing due to the different fitness regimes that did not agree with their fitness levels or age.

Putting together my experiences, the advice I had learned, and what I'd been hearing from others, I discovered a way to help the elderly with fitness routines that developed and enhanced strength to ensure that their bodies continued in the same state as their younger years.

This chapter is not just about words that are on a piece of paper, it's about possibilities. As you get to step forward moving into the world of strength training through your golden years you are making an effort to get into a world of transformation. This is a place where your resilience and vitality will take center stage. Let's dive into the heart of the matter and explore why strength matters so profoundly in this incredible and new phase of life.

The Importance of Being Strong and Healthy in Your Golden Years

It's sad to realize, but this is a world that celebrates youth and all of the benefits that come from being young and healthy. This doesn't mean that being a senior or an elder means that you won't be celebrated or people look at you differently; however, people do feel that we can and should allow our bodies to maintain our strength and health well into our senior years. It isn't that it is something impossible to achieve. The way that we choose to live our lives, our lifestyle choices, the decisions we make, the foods that we eat, and the activities that we participate in, all of these come to revitalize and boost or diminish our health and strength.

Remember, your strength is timeless. This is not about lifting heavy and massive weights or becoming a superhero, someone who's doing things that are unimaginable and impossible—it's about having the power to live your life on your terms. It's about living life well into your senior years without needing to follow the natural and usual process that most of the elderly have been accustomed to in the past. Why is this important (Butcher, 2023)?

Maintaining Independence Throughout Any Age

Just imagine it, this isn't about your muscles—It's about your ability to walk with purpose and determination, the ability to stand up tall and sit up. It's how you embrace every moment in life with confidence—knowing that you can and do what you need to. It's a type of passport to maintain an independent and fulfilling lifestyle.

Now, imagine if this strength that enabled you to stand and walk was taken away from you. Your independence would be gone. You would need either a family member or a caregiver to help you with fulfilling and completing simple tasks like helping you bathe in the morning, getting dressed, brushing your teeth, eating your breakfast, and every other activity you need to do from there.

Preventing Common Health Issues

Your strength is your ally against the most common adversities of aging. This includes health issues like heart troubles, diabetes, and osteoporosis. This isn't only about building muscle, it has nothing to do with what your physique looks like, it's all about building resilience against the potential hurdles that will come your way as soon as you begin the senior years of life.

Try to picture a life where you choose that sedentary lifestyle. Along with doing nothing comes the potential to develop serious chronic health conditions. Now, imagine not being able to do much on your own and care for yourself including the fact that your health is deteriorating and your body is in pain.

The Benefits and Difference of Strength Training—Its Unique Nature

Strength training is a bit different when compared to other types of exercises. It almost mirrors a secret potion that can help stimulate your muscle growth and enhance your bone density all while helping to keep you moving fluidly. It's entirely based on functional strength that helps to continue with real-life movements without any stress strain or injury to your body.

Let's look at the benefits of strength training as a ripple effect on your overall well-being.

This training boosts your overall health by

- revving up your metabolism. It's almost like you're giving your body's engine a boost. You are helping to manage your weight effectively. You might even ask the question: Who would have thought that lifting a few weights could make such a difference?
- healing your heart. Cardiovascular health isn't just improved by doing cardio but it's about having a heart that beats strong and strength training doesn't just help pump iron, it's about pumping life into your heart as well. This isn't about muscles, it's about what happens on the inside as well.
- boosting mood and mental health. With strength training, endorphins are released and this is a magical mood-boosting chemical that will help paint your days with positivity. This isn't just about physical strength, it's about fortifying your mental fortress.
- enhancing your cognitive function. This type of training isn't just about getting strong on the outside, it's also about sharpening your cognitive abilities and keeping your mental faculties agile and sharp.

Overcoming Common Challenges: Immobility, Muscle Fatigue, and Weakness

As you age, some hurdles and burdens will try to drag you down. Obviously, these are common and natural side effects of getting older as your body begins to deteriorate.

Why We Face These Issues

- As we age, there are quite a few changes that take place naturally in our physical bodies. These changes vary from person to person but most people tend to experience (Mayo Clinic, 2022)
- muscle atrophy and loss of muscle mass. Sarcopenia is an age-related loss of muscle mass that can begin as early as the mid-thirties and this issue becomes more pronounced with age. The reason why this happens is because of a decrease in the number and the size of muscle fibers. Certain factors like reduced protein synthesis, hormonal changes, and inadequate dietary protein intake can all come together and contribute to this condition.

- reduced muscle strength occurs as aging adults tend to experience a decline in the efficiency of their nervous system's control over muscle contractions. This can result in reduced muscle strength and coordination. Again with aging, there is a certain shift from the fast-twitch muscle fibers which are responsible for your exclusive power to slow-twitch fibers which are responsible for endurance. This change leads to a decrease in muscle strength but increased endurance.
- decreased mobility occurs as there is a loss of joint flexibility and increased stiffness because of the changes in the cartilage and synovial fluid within the joints. This issue can limit the range of motion that you have, as well as make your movements much more challenging. Again, another issue is reduced bone density which causes osteoporosis. This is a common condition and occurs as a result of weakened bones. This increases the risk of fractures. This can reduce your willingness to move freely and engage in physical activities.
- muscle fatigue occurs when mitochondria—your energy-producing cells—become less efficient with age. This issue makes it easier for you to experience muscle fatigue during physical activity as your muscles struggle to produce sufficient energy. There is also a decline in aerobic capacity since aging causes your body to become less efficient in utilizing oxygen during exercise.
- inactivity and lifestyle factors like living a sedentary lifestyle, inadequate intake of essential nutrients, and poor nutrition, as well as chronic illnesses can exacerbate muscle weakness and inability. They can worsen your muscle atrophy and cause you to feel weak. Eventually, all of these issues come together to reduce your mobility and muscle strength.
- finally, psychological factors like the fear of falling increase. As we age we become more cautious to avoid falling which can further limit our physical activity and lead to muscle weakness.

As we age we should understand that it is a highly individualized process and not everyone will experience the same issues or to the same extent. With regular physical activity, a balanced diet, and proper healthcare, we can help mitigate some of these effects as we get to maintain functional independence in our later years. Additionally, targeted exercise programs, like strength training exercises, can help improve muscle strength and mobility as you age. So yes, we will face issues as we age but fear not because we've got solutions to them.

These exercises gently challenge your muscles and show them that they can rise above fatigue and become stronger than ever. Remember that weakness is not a life sentence; it's more of a challenge waiting to be conquered. The strength training exercises that you will find in the following chapters will guide you into the path of rebuilding your strength one step at a time, one movement at a time. Before we get to look into strength training in more detail, let's just debunk some of the myths about strength training so that you can take off on this journey with the right frame of mind. Jumping into something without expecting any results can lead you to zero results. For almost every aspect or situation, we should always try to keep a positive mindset so that we get to absorb the most benefits out of whatever we are doing. By choosing to remain negative, your body and mind will reject the idea of whatever you are doing or sabotage you in some way or another as you think that there is no need to practice a specific activity.

Debunking Myths About Strength Training as We Age

Let's tackle those myths that might have held you back.

Myth: Seniors are too old for strength training.

Fact: The reality is that age isn't a barrier, it's more of a canvas waiting to be painted with strength. There are low-impact exercises suitable for every age group.

Myth: Strength training will lead you to bulky muscles.

Fact: Strength training empowers your body. Bulky muscles can be only obtained once you introduce higher levels of protein intake into your diet.

Myth: You need to train at a gym as it's impossible to train without weights.

Fact: The truth is that strength training can be done safely and effectively at home. We will look at some strength training activities where you see just how exactly you can do these exercises at home.

Myth: Strength training is very dangerous for seniors.

Fact: The reality is that when any sort of exercise is done in the correct form, it is safe and immensely beneficial. The same is true for strength training.

Myth: Only young people benefit from strength training and older people should focus more on doing tai chi and meditation techniques instead.

Fact: The truth is that strength training benefits are ageless. Your golden years deserve gold-standard care.

Myth: Strength training increases the risk of injury as it is a very difficult type of exercise.

Fact: The truth is that with proper guidance and technique tips, you can minimize the risk of injury. Also, there are modifications that you could incorporate into the exercises if you feel that you are unable to practice them as is.

Myth: Strength training is time-consuming and requires heavy weights.

Fact: You can participate in brief sessions which yield impressive results. It's more about quality over quantity. Also, resistance can come in many forms and you can choose what suits you best. You do not need to invest in any heavy weights.

As we come to the end of this chapter just allow that excitement to take hold of you. You are on the brink of something incredible, strengthening your body and embracing the beauty of your golden years to bring you closer to a younger, more vibrant you.

Let's turn the page and continue this adventure together.

Chapter 2

THE SCIENCE AND BENEFITS OF STRENGTH AND RESISTANCE TRAINING

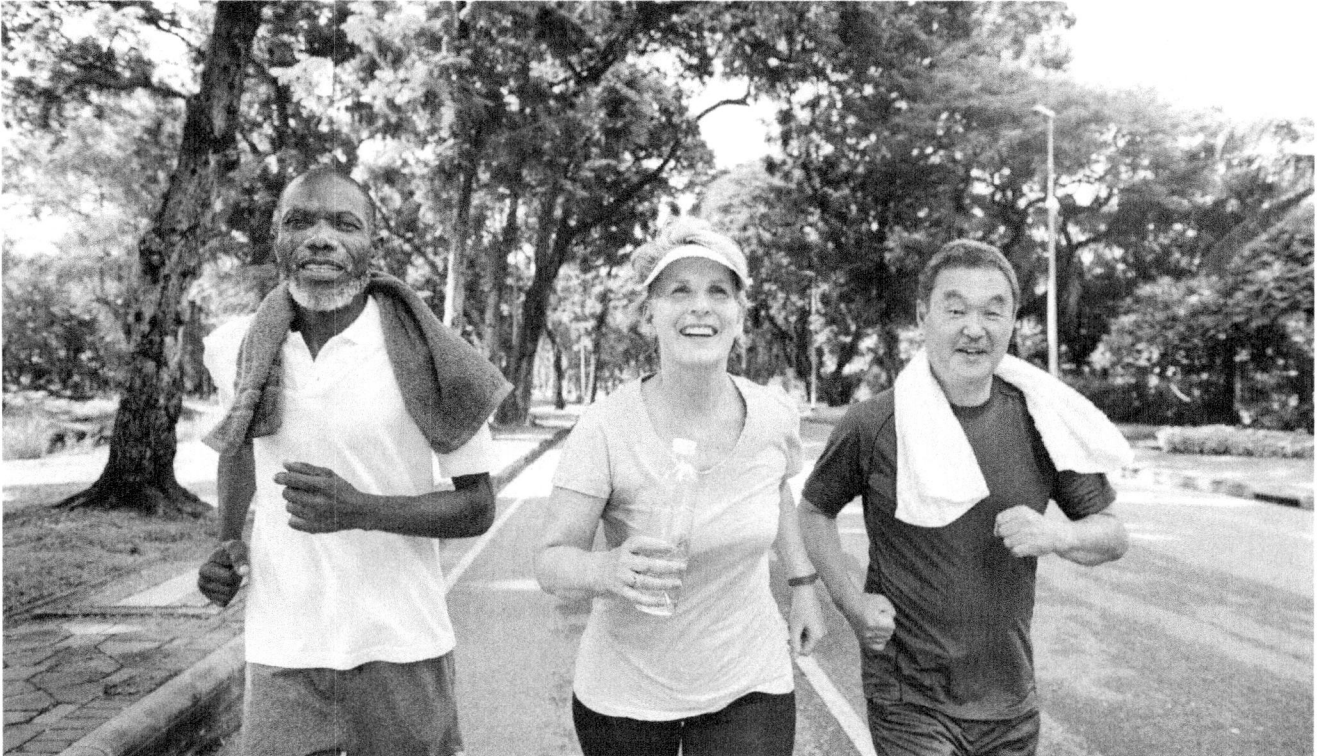

Now it's time to dive deep into the world of strength and resistance training. As I usually tell my class at the community center, I like to keep it simple for you to understand quickly so that you can identify just what exactly you need to know about the exercises and how they can benefit you as you get ready for the movements. Let's get started.

Strength and Resistance Training

Both of these exercises are sort of like superheroes in the exercise category. They help with building muscle and enabling you to become stronger, despite whatever age group you fall into. The best part is that they can be done at any age and you can start despite low fitness levels.

Strength training is a type of exercise where you use your muscles to lift, push, or pull against resistance. This resistance can come from almost anything, like weights, dumbbells, or even your own body weight. Try to think of it as though you are using your body to do a certain activity while being pushed or pulled against it by the force of gravity. Imagine you are doing push-ups or lifting weights at the gym, that's strength training. Seeing as how simple it is, let's move on to the next exercise, which is almost similar to strength training.

Resistance training is often referred to as the cousin of strength training. Here, it's all about using resistance to make your muscles work harder. It can be done with exercise bands or even water. Try to imagine yourself doing leg lifts in a pool; that's resistance training.

A Historical Perspective

Let's go back in time a little bit. Strength training has been around for ages and over the years, like everything else, it has evolved. Back in ancient Greece, athletes used to lift heavy stones and compete in strength contests. It was around the 19th century when strong men like Eugene Sandow became famous for their incredible strength feats (Heffernan, 2014). However, it's not that you need to become a strong man or an ancient Greek to benefit from strength training. This type of exercise is for everyone and I'll show you exactly how to do it so that it is gentle and low-impact. This basically means that it's safe and simple enough to do for you, no matter what age group you fall into or how strong or weak you currently are.

The Importance of Strength Training

We have already looked at the fact that strength training isn't just for those who are interested in becoming heavyweight champions or athletes. It's also not the type of exercise that's just done if you want to build your muscles to look like Mr. or Miss Olympia.

Strength is vital, as it

- helps you maintain your muscle mass, keeping you strong and independent. Always keep in mind that your muscles naturally become weaker with age.
- boosts metabolism by building muscles, which helps you burn more calories. This is a great way for you to maintain a healthy weight
- enhancing bone health. As you age, your bones become weaker. Strength training is the secret agent for your bones. It helps make them denser and stronger, which will aid in decreasing the risk of developing osteoporosis and fracturing should you fall.
- improves cardiovascular health. Strength training doesn't just help your muscles and bones; it's also great for your heart. It helps lower blood pressure while reducing the risk of developing heart disease.
- makes it easier to complete day-to-day tasks. For example, it'll be much easier for you to carry groceries from the car to the house, so it'll be easier for you to

play with your grandchildren and carry them. It will also be very easy to get off a chair, walk up that stairwell, and go for that daily jog.

- After a few times of engaging in strength training activities, you will notice that you develop a liking for them. It doesn't have to be a sure thing; it's more of a fun activity that you get to do to replace a sedentary lifestyle.

Understanding the Science Behind Strength Training

You may be wondering just why exactly strength training has such a profound effect and impact on our bodies, especially as we age. Well, now it's time to uncover the fascinating science behind these exercises. We will break it down from complex to bite-sized so that it's easy to grasp and once you understand the why behind strength training, you'll be even more motivated to reap its benefits.

Muscle Physiology

A great way to look at your muscles is by imagining them as your body's engine. They help you move, lift things, and even smile. Let's take a quick peek at how they work.

Muscles are made up of tiny fibers; some are fast and powerful, while others are slow and steady. Strength training works on both of these types of fibers, helping to make them stronger. When you begin to lift a weight or do a push-up, your brain will send a signal to your muscles telling them to contract or squeeze. This is basically how you get to move things. After a strength training session, your muscles will feel a bit sore. This is a sign to show you that they are growing and getting stronger.

Progressive Overload

Try to imagine carrying the same grocery bags with the same weight often. Your muscles won't get any stronger but they will be able to endure this movement. To make them grow, you will need to challenge them more.

Progressive overload is the secret source of strength training. This means that you are gradually increasing the weight or resistance while you exercise and your muscles get stronger. It's almost the same as leveling up in a video game.

Adaptation is when your muscles learn to adapt to the demands of life. When you lift heavier weights or do more repetitions of exercises, your muscles will be saying that they need to get stronger for this and that's how you build more muscle over time.

Now, before we move on, it's important that you understand that muscles are built on protein. As you exercise and put strain and pressure on your muscles, there may be microfiber tears. This is a natural part of exercising, where they grow stronger. To get your muscles to grow and become much stronger than they were previously, you will need to incorporate protein into your diet. You can try adding protein powders as a snack or having protein bars on the go. This protein will then be used for the repair and growth of your muscle fibers.

Neuromuscular Adaptations

Strength training isn't just about your muscles; it's also about your brain and nerves working together with your muscles.

As you train, your brain gets better at telling your muscles what to do. It enhances your neuromuscular coordination.

Another great benefit is that your coordination is improved as you are better able to control your body. This will help your movements become more smooth, your balance will improve, and there will be a greater reduction in the risk of falls.

Hormonal Responses

Our bodies have some special hormones that play a role in strength training.

The growth hormone is important as it helps repair and grow your muscles. It's almost like a repair crew for your muscle fibers. They are released when you lift weights.

Testosterone is a hormone that both men and women have. Men have a higher level than women, but this hormone is very important when it comes to building muscle and strength. Strength training can increase your body's testosterone levels naturally.

Nutrition and Recovery

Now it's time to talk about what you eat and how you rest. This is very essential when it comes to your strength training journey.

When it comes to food, your body needs the right type of fuel to build and repair muscles. Protein is like the building blocks for muscles so you will need to ensure that you are getting enough in your diet. You can incorporate protein-rich foods into your diet.

- Lean meats like pork tenderloin, lean beef, turkey breast, and chicken breast
- Seafood like salmon, tilapia, shrimp, tuna, and cod
- Poultry like chicken, turkey, and duck
- Eggs; whole eggs, or egg whites
- Dairy or dairy alternatives like Greek yogurt, cottage cheese, milk, which includes plant-based options like almond milk and soy milk, and cheese, which should be moderately consumed,
- Legumes like chickpeas, black peas, kidney beans, and lentils

- Nuts and seeds like chia seeds, pumpkin seeds, sunflower seeds, almonds, and peanuts.
- Tofu
- Tempeh
- Quinoa
- Wild rice
- Protein supplements like whey protein, pea protein, and hemp protein powders added to smoothies or recipes.

When it comes to protein content, remember that it varies among different brands and cooking methods. It's also important that you balance your protein intake with a well-rounded diet that includes vegetables, fruits, whole grains, and healthy fats to ensure that you are getting a wide range of nutrients for optimal health.

When it comes to recovery, you will need to incorporate some resting time after every strength training session. Remember that your muscles need time to recover and grow. Therefore, getting enough sleep, staying hydrated, and managing your stress levels are key components of recovery.

Now you have all the knowledge you need about the science behind strength training. You understand now that it isn't just about lifting weights, it's more about how your muscles, nerves, hormones, and diet all come together to make you stronger and healthier. Let's move on to discovering how strength training can be gentle and accessible to everyone regardless of their age or fitness level.

How Strength Training Can Still Be Gentle, Low-Impact and Accessible To Everyone

Strength training is a type of exercise that isn't just for any specific person, it's for everyone. And it's essential to make it accessible and inclusive. Let's just explore the ways that we can ensure that you and everyone can benefit from it, no matter what your age is or your physical condition.

Adaptable Exercise Modalities

There are a variety of options that you could use that would suit your different preferences and needs. Some of this includes:

- Bodyweight exercises where no fancy equipment is needed. You use your body as the weight and resistance for exercises. Some examples include planks, push-ups, and squats.
- Resistance bands are stretchy bands that provide resistance for your muscles. They are very lightweight and portable, and they are great for gentle strength training.

- Free weights like dumbbells or kettlebells come in a variety of sizes, which allows you to choose the right weight for your fitness level. As you become stronger, you can increase your weight.

Low-impact Strength Training

It's important that you do not worry about strength training being difficult for you, especially if you have joint issues or mobility limitations. These exercises can still be gentle enough and safe for you.

- There are low-impact exercises you could choose from that put less stress on your joints. These include seated leg lifts, seated rows, or wall push-ups.
- Swimming is a great low-impact exercise since the water provides resistance without any impact, which makes it an excellent option for strength training for those with joint issues and mobility limitations.
- Tai chi is an ancient practice that combines gentle movements and strength-building to help you improve your balance and flexibility.

Incorporating Modifications

Strength training isn't a one-size-fits-all approach. You can modify exercises to suit your fitness level and physical abilities. Modifications include:

- Reducing the intensity of each exercise, for example, you could start out with lighter weights or fewer repetitions and gradually increase as you become stronger.
- Using support from a wall, chair, or balance aid can help you maintain stability during exercises.
- Consulting a trainer or a fitness professional who can tailor strength training exercises to suit your specific needs.

Accessible Facilities

Accessible facilities and adaptive equipment can make a big difference when it comes to your exercise routines and physical fitness levels. Some of these facilities have

- wheelchair-friendly gym that has ramps and accessible equipment.
- adaptive tools or specialized equipment like seated leg presses or hand crank machines that can cater to various ranges of abilities.
- inclusive classes are offered at specific community centers that provide inclusive strength training classes for those with various health needs.

Now it's time for us to move on to why you, as a senior, can greatly benefit from strength training.

Seniors and the Benefits of Strength Training

This type of exercise can be a game-changer for you as a senior, as it promotes your overall health and well-being. Let's delve deeper into just how exactly it can be beneficial for you (Mayer et al., 2011).

Healthy Aging

As we age, the natural process involves muscle weakening, but strength training can help reverse the effects.

It helps preserve muscle mass by fighting muscle loss. This helps you maintain your strength and independence as you get older. It also enhances your bone density, as strong muscles also support healthy bones, which reduces your risk of fractures and osteoporosis.

Improved Mobility

Another issue that comes along as we age is that our joints and bones can change as well. Strength training, as we have already seen, isn't just about our muscles. It's about movement as well.

Joint mobility is improved and this can reduce stiffness as you participate in exercises like leg lifts and squats. Strength training also enhances your balance, which can reduce the risk of falls which can be very important when it comes to an aging adult.

Managing Chronic Conditions

Strength training also offers benefits for chronic health conditions.

We have already looked at how it is beneficial for strengthening your bones, which reduces the risk of osteoporosis and fractures. Regular strength training can improve your blood sugar levels, which will reduce the risk of developing diabetes or help manage it. With these exercises, improving the muscles around effective joints can reduce pain and improve your function, which reduces the risk of developing or maintaining arthritis.

Cognitive Benefits

Strength training isn't just for your body; it's also very beneficial to your mind as well. It is a brain booster as it enhances cognitive function and memory.

Psychological Well-being

Strength training also acts as a mood lifter, as it reduces stress and anxiety by triggering the release of endorphins. Regular involvement and strength-training exercises also help boost your mood and combat feelings of depression.

Social Aspects

Exercise doesn't have to be a chore; it can be fun and even a social activity.

You can join a strength training class, as this is a great way to meet new people and stay motivated. Some communities may offer strength training programs that are tailored to your needs.

Always keep in mind that strength training isn't just about lifting weights and building muscles; it's about enhancing your quality of life, regardless of your age or fitness level. We have looked at the world of strength training, covering the science, adaptability, incredible benefits, and how it is one of the greatest exercise options for you as a senior. Now, in the next chapter, we are going to look at some strength training exercises that you could try out to get yourself in shape. Regardless of your age or current fitness level, you can benefit from training exercises, so don't hesitate to start exploring the world of strength and resistance training today.

Chapter 3

50-ILLUSTRATED STRENGTH AND RESISTANCE TRAINING

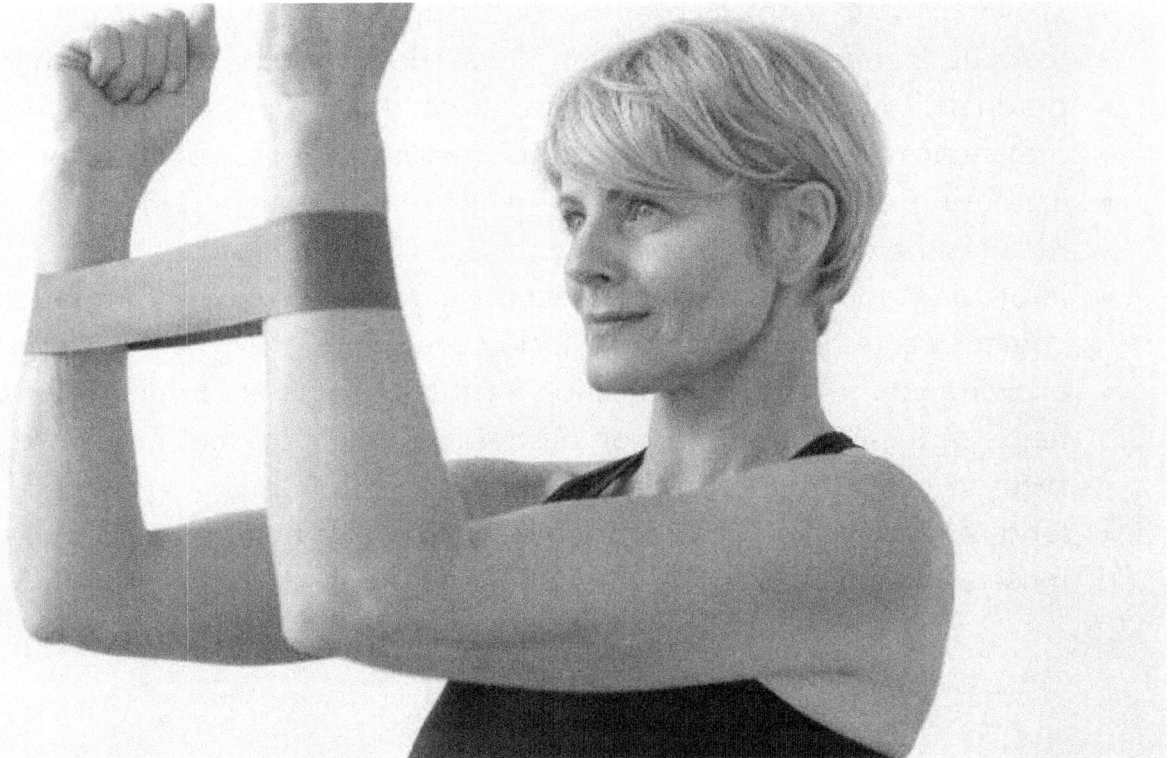

In this chapter we are going to look at a wide range of strength and resistance training exercises. Each one will be presented with detailed instructions accompanied by an illustration to help you familiarize yourself with just how exactly you need to position your body and how to perform the exercise in the proper form. The exercises are categorized into different difficulty levels to ensure that there's something for you no matter what fitness level you are currently at. You also get to have modification suggestions to help lessen the strain or pressure of each exercise. Not to wait any longer let's get to it.

Warm-up Exercises

Before we move into the exercises, it's important that you understand what warm-up exercises are. This is the first group of movements that you should do to get your muscles and body prepared for the activities you are about to engage in. There are a variety of benefits that come from warm-ups which include

- reducing the risk of muscle strains and other injuries as your body is more prepared for intense physical activity.

- improving the elasticity and flexibility of your muscles which enhances your range of motion and makes it less likely for your muscles to be overstretched or damaged during exercise.
- warming up your body, causing your blood vessels to dilate which allows for more oxygen and nutrients to reach your muscles.
- allowing you to mentally prepare for the upcoming physical activity which helps to focus, increase your awareness of your body, and boost your confidence.
- gradually raise your body temperature which improves the efficiency of metabolic reactions in your body. This leads to better overall performance.
- increasing the heat in your body which eases your muscles into action and reduces the sensation of stiffness.
- improving your reflexes and reaction times which is very important when it comes to activities that require quick movements.
- allowing you to mentally transition from a resting state to an active one, which helps reduce anxiety and nervousness making you feel more prepared and focused.
- long-term benefits such as improved flexibility and reduced risk of chronic muscle and joint issues.

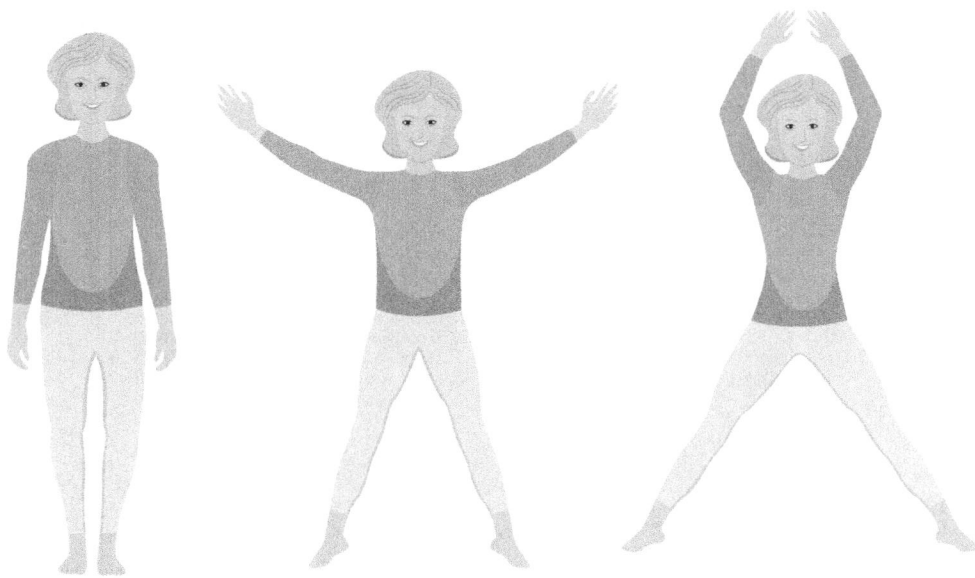

- Start by standing straight, your arms hanging loosely at your side and your feet close together.
- Begin at a slow pace and gradually increase the intensity to get your heart rate up.
- Focus on controlled breathing.
- Jump up with your feet extending outwards as you land on them with your hands moving up above your head.
- Jump again, this time your feet and arms returning to your start position.
- Repeat 20 jumps.

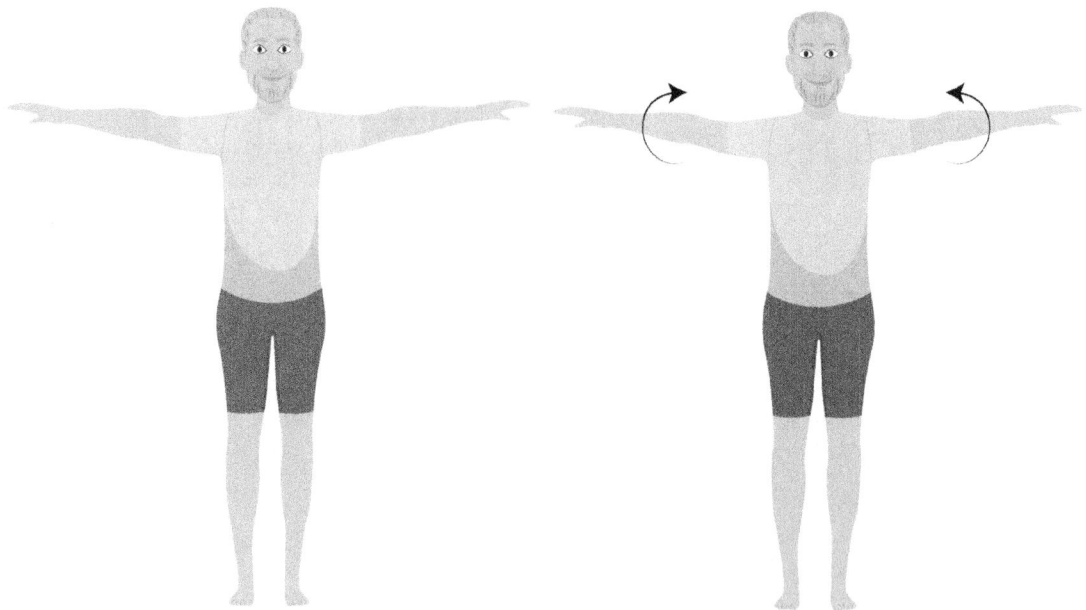

- Stand on a flat surface.
- Extend your arms out towards your sides at shoulder height.
- Begin rotating your arms in small circles clockwise, increasing the size gradually for 15 seconds.
- Keep your breathing controlled, back straight, and shoulders back.
- Bring your arms to a stop and then repeat the motion in the opposite direction.

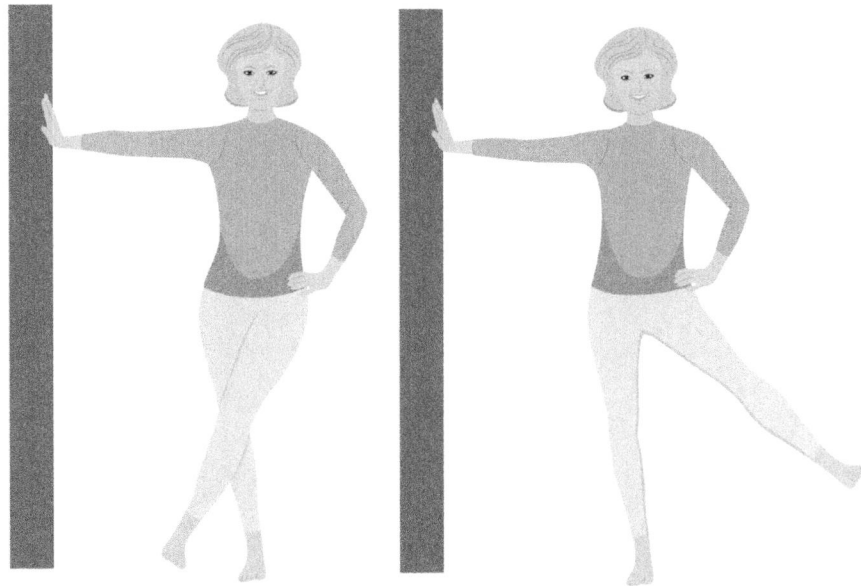

- Use a wall or a railing to hold onto for balance.
- Place your arm against the wall.
- Swing the leg away from the wall left and right and then forward and backward in a controlled manner.
- Keep your breathing controlled.
- Your back should be straight and shoulders back.
- Repeat this 15 times then stop and turn in the other direction.
- Repeat the same motion on the other side.

Now it's time to move into the exercises.

Strength and Resistance Exercises

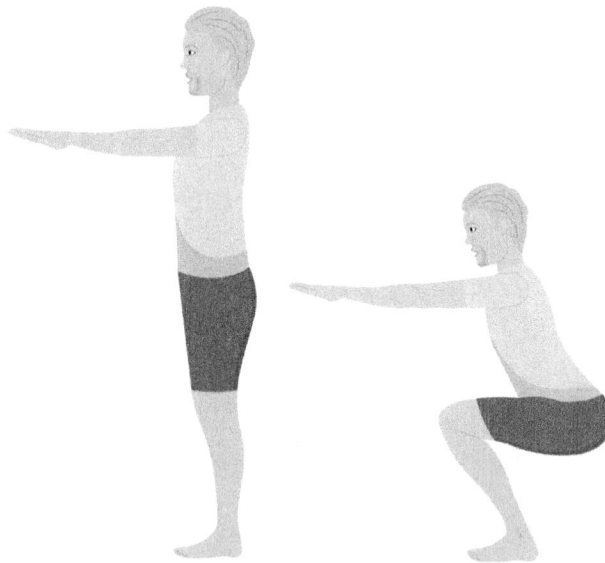

- Begin by standing up straight with your feet hip-width apart, toes pointing slightly outward.
- Place your hands on your hips or you could extend them out in front of you for balance.
- As you get ready, engage your core muscles by pulling your belly button towards your spine.
- Maintain controlled breathing.
- Begin the movements of the squat by pushing your hips back as if you are sitting in a chair to lower your body gently by bending your knees while keeping your back straight.
- Keep your knees aligned with your feet. They should not go beyond your toes.
- Go as low as you can but no more than is comfortable for you.
- Try to keep your thighs parallel to the ground.
- Hold the position at the bottom of the squat before pushing through your heels to stand back up as you straighten your legs.
- Return to your start position.
- Stand tall with your hips fully extended.
- Repeat this exercise 10 to 15 times, 2 to 3 sets.

You can modify this exercise by using a sturdy chair or a bench for support. Stand in front of the chair as you lower yourself down into the squat position, and lightly touch the chair with your bottom before standing back up. This will help reduce the depth of the squat.

You could also perform a shallow squat instead of going as low; you can only go part way down until you build strength and confidence.

You could also use a sturdy surface like a countertop or wall for balancing and assistance.

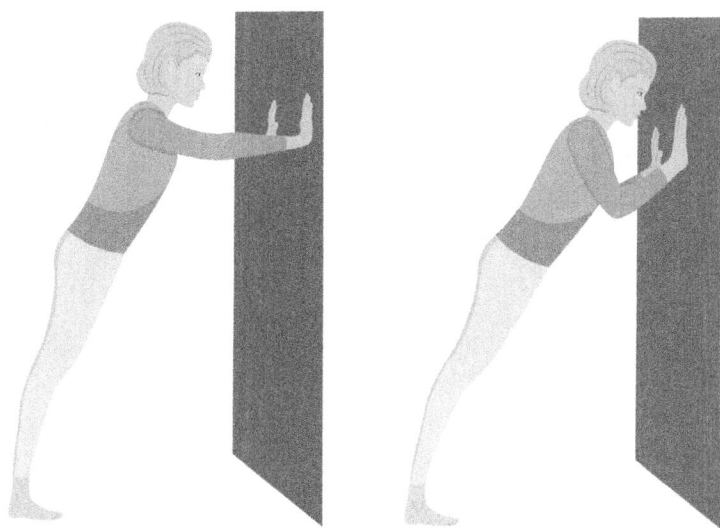

- Stand up straight facing a sturdy wall.
- Your feet should be hip-width apart.
- Place your hands on the wall at shoulder height slightly wider than shoulder-width apart.
- Your fingers should be pointing upwards.
- Step back slightly, a few feet away from the wall to create an angle with your body.
- Try to keep your body aligned as you begin to engage your core muscles by pulling your belly button in toward your spine.
- Bend your elbows and lower your chest wall to wall.
- Go as close as possible to the wall as you can without straining.
- Your arms should be comfortable and there should be no pain.
- Stay in this position for a moment at the bottom of the push-up.
- Slowly push through your palms to straighten your arms and return to the starting position.

- Repeat the exercise 10 to 15 times, 3 to 5 sets.
- Maintain a controlled pace throughout the exercise.

If the exercise is a bit difficult you can modify it by adjusting your distance from the wall. The closer you stand the less challenging it will be. First start with a greater distance and gradually decrease it as you build strength.

You could also use a higher surface to perform the push-ups like a sturdy table or countertop to reduce the angle and make it easier for you.

Gradually you can work yourself towards doing full wall push-ups and then moving from the wall to the floor.

PLANK | *DIFFICULTY–INTERMEDIATE*

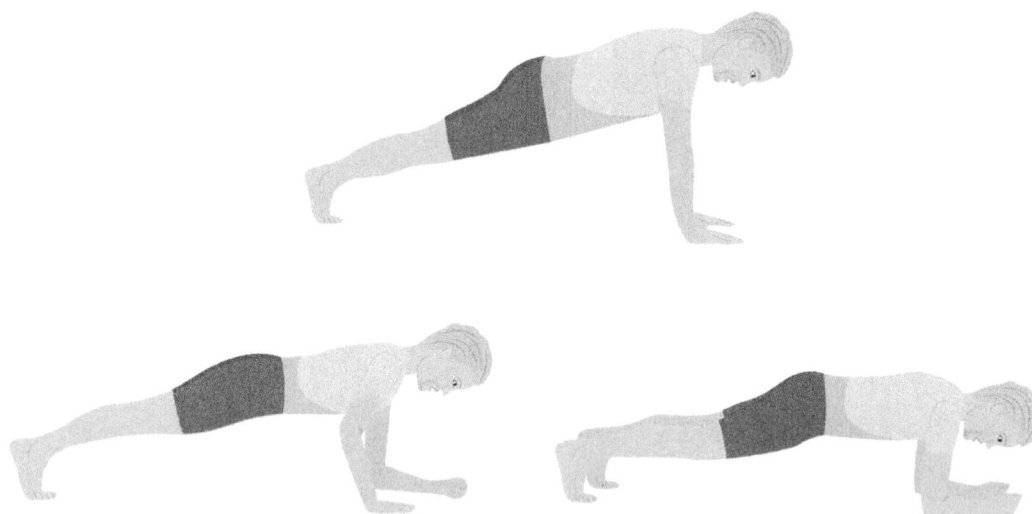

- You will first need to get into a push-up position.
- Your hands should be shoulder-width apart.
- Your elbows should be bent at 90-degree angles and your forearms should rest on the ground.
- Remember to keep your body in a straight line from your head to your heels.
- Engage your core muscles as you practice deep breathing.
- Your shoulders should be directly above your elbows and your hands should be flat on the ground.
- Hold this position for a few seconds as you maintain a straight body while keeping your head in a neutral position.
- Focus on keeping your breath steady and even throughout the exercise.
- Try to hold the plank for 10 to 30 seconds. As you progress you can increase the duration.

- Repeat this exercise 2 to 3 times.

If it is too difficult, bend your knees and touch them against the ground. So instead of using the push-up position, you will start on your knees with your forearms on the ground as you maintain a straight line from your head to your knees.

You could also use an elevated surface where you place your forearms on a sturdy surface like a bench or table as you keep your body straight to reduce the intensity.

Another way to modify this exercise is to start with shorter durations and gradually work your way up.

SEATED LEG-RAISES | *DIFFICULTY—BEGINNER*

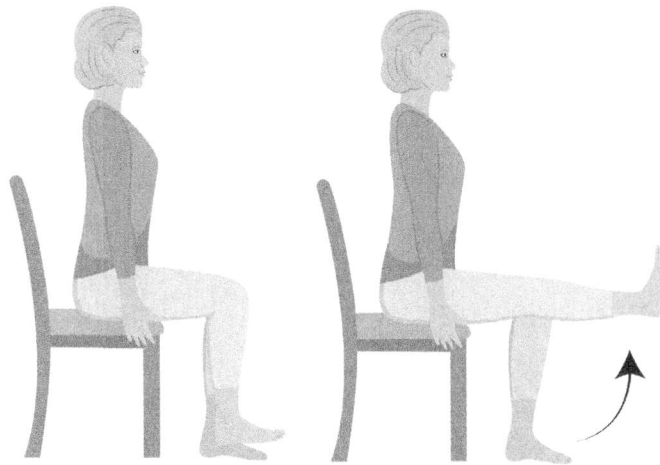

- Begin by sitting on a sturdy chair.
- Your back should be straight.
- Your feet should be flat on the ground and your hands should be resting on your thighs.
- Engage your core muscles as you begin deep belly breathing. Imagine pulling your belly button toward your spine.
- Remember to keep your back against the chair's backrest for support.
- Gently lift your right leg off the ground, extending it straight in front of you.
- Hold this position for a few seconds before bringing it down.
- As you hold, focus on using your hip flexor muscles.
- Lower your leg back down to the ground.
- Repeat the movement with the other leg.
- Continue alternating your legs for the desired number of repetitions.
- Perform 8 to 15 leg raises on each side with 2 to 5 sets.

To modify, you can start with smaller leg raises.

You could also hold on to the armrest of the chair or the sides for added stability and support.

You can perform this exercise at a much slower pace to maintain control and reduce its intensity.

BENT-OVER DUMBBELL ROWS | *DIFFICULTY–INTERMEDIATE*

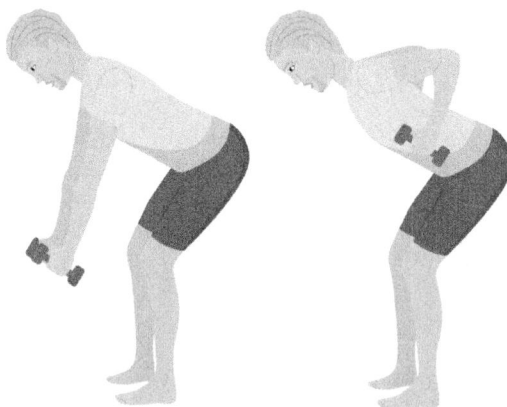

- Start by standing up straight with your feet at hip-width apart.
- You should be holding a dumbbell in each hand with your arms fully extended down in front of you.
- Begin to engage your core muscles as you pull your belly button to your spine.
- Hinge at your hips, do not be stiff.
- Bend your knees slightly and lean forward as you keep your back straight.
- You could also try ensuring that your bottom is pushed out so that the spine is not arching.
- Let your arms hang straight down in front of you with your palms facing your thighs.
- Start the motion of the exercise which is referred to as a roll by bending your elbows and pulling the dumbbells up towards your hips, while you squeeze your shoulder blades together.
- Keep your elbows close to your body.
- Pause for a moment at the top of the roll.
- Slowly begin to lower the dumbbells back down to the starting position and fully extend your arms.
- Maintain a controlled pace throughout the exercise.
- Ensure that your body is aligned and in a proper form.
- Repeat 8 to 10 rows on each arm.
- Perform 2 to 5 sets.

To make this exercise easier you can start with lighter dumbbells to reduce the resistance.

You can also perform it with your back against a wall for some added stability.

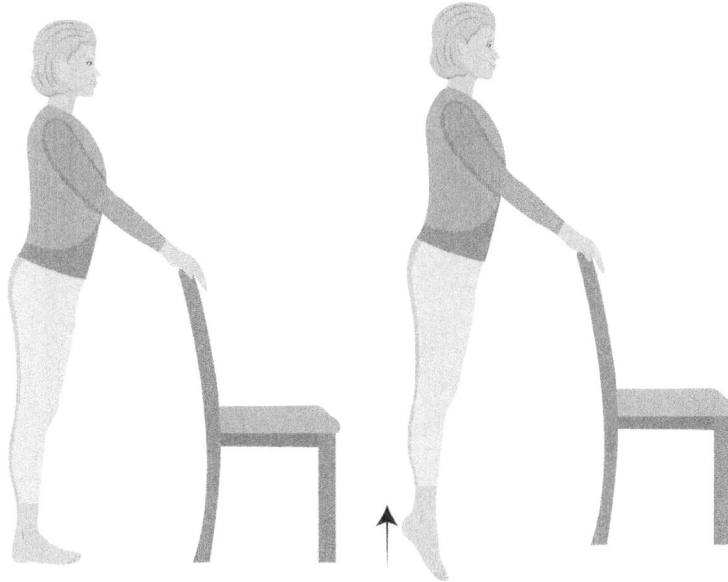

- Begin by standing tall. Your feet should be hip-width apart.
- Make sure to position yourself near a wall or a sturdy surface that you can hold onto for balance if needed.
- Your back must be straight, your shoulders relaxed as your core is engaged with deep breathing.
- Slowly begin to raise your heels off the ground as you push through the balls of your feet.
- Continue lifting your heels as high as you can go, comfortably.
- Focus on contracting your calf muscles.
- Hold this position for a few seconds as you feel that stretch in your calves.
- Lower your heels back down slowly to your starting position.
- Repeat this movement 8 to 15 times.
- Perform 2 to 5 sets.

To modify and make this exercise easier you can perform it while holding onto a sturdy chair or countertop for some added support.

You could also do partial calf raises where you lift your heels only a few inches off the ground.

You could also use a wall for stability.

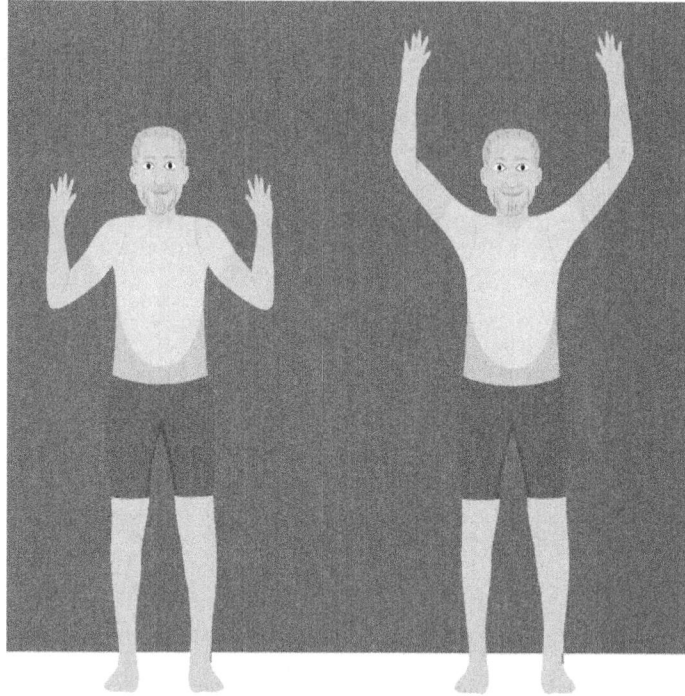

- Stand up straight with your back against the wall.
- Your heels, buttocks, upper back, and head must all be in contact with the wall.
- Your feet should be hip-width apart and a few inches away from the wall.
- Begin by extending your arms straight out to your sides.
- Your palms should be facing forward and your fingers should be pointing upwards.
- Slide your arms up along the wall as you bring your hands overhead without allowing them to lose contact with the wall behind you.
- Raise your arms as high as you can without lifting your shoulders off the wall.
- At the top, your arms should form a y-shape above your head.
- Slowly bring your arms back down to the starting position.
- Remember to maintain contact with the wall.
- Repeat this movement 10 to 15 times.
- Perform 4 to 8 sets.

You can modify this exercise to make it easier by starting with smaller movements, for example, moving your arms from shoulder level just slightly above your shoulder level.

You could also use a soft surface like a padded or foam roll against a wall which will provide you with more comfort and support.

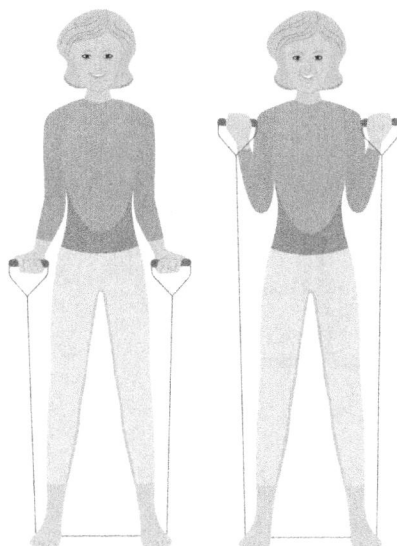

- Start by choosing a resistance band. Keep in mind that the toughness of the band is what determines the difficulty level of this exercise.
- Step on the center of the resistance band with both your feet.
- Ensure that the band is secure under the arches of your feet.
- Stand with your feet hip-width apart.
- Bend your knees lightly.
- Keep your core engaged with deep breaths.
- Begin by holding the handles or the ends of the resistance band in each hand with your arms fully extended and your palms facing forward.
- Keep your elbows close to your sides throughout the exercise.
- Begin the curl as you bend your elbows.
- Bring your hands towards your shoulders while keeping your upper arms stationary.
- Try to keep your body aligned, your head, back, and legs should be in a straight line.
- Squeeze your biceps at the top of the curl.
- Slowly lower your hands back to the starting position as you fully extend your arms.
- Maintain a controlled pace.
- Focus on your biceps throughout the movements.
- Repeat this exercise 8 to 15 times and perform 2 to 5 sets.

If it's too difficult for you to lift up your arms with the resistance band you can choose one with lower tension to reduce the intensity. You can also perform this exercise while seated on a sturdy chair to provide you with better stability.

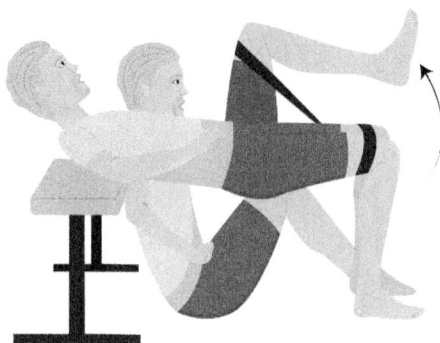

- This exercise will require you to own a resistance band and bench.
- Begin the exercise by using the resistance band that is placed around your knees.
- Lean back against the bench while sitting on the floor.
- You will then need to lift your bottom up ensuring that your upper back is resting on the bench while your lower body is suspended over the ground and your legs are firmly planted on the ground.
- Your knees should be bent at a 90-degree angle.
- Ensure that the band is secured.
- Engage your core muscles. Slowly extend one leg in front of you while keeping the other foot firm on the floor.
- Hold this position for a moment.
- Feel the resistance from the band.
- Slowly return your foot to the starting position.
- Repeat the movement with the other leg.
- Continue alternating 8 to 15 times with each leg.
- Perform 3 to 5 sets.

If this exercise is too difficult for you, you can do it while lying down on the floor.

You could also choose a resistance band that has less tension to reduce the intensity.

You can also begin with partial extensions where you lift your foot only a few inches off the ground.

You could hold onto the sides of the bench to aid with stability and support.

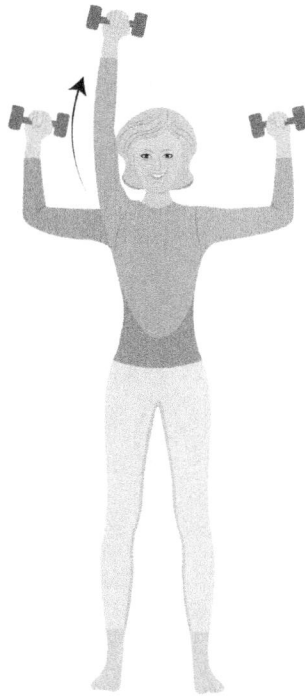

- Start by moving into position, standing tall.
- Your feet should be hip-width apart with your knees slightly bent.
- You should have a comfortable weighted dumbbell in each hand—you can use food cans if you like.
- Start the motions by holding the dumbbells at shoulder height with your palms facing forward.
- Your elbows should be bent at 90-degree angles and your arms should be parallel to the ground.
- Engage your core muscles with deep belly breathing as you pull your belly button towards your spine.
- Keep your back straight, your shoulders back, and your chest up.
- Press or lift the dumbbell overhead by extending your arms fully while exhaling
- Straighten your arms completely without locking your elbows.
- Hold this position for a few seconds as you focus on your shoulder muscles.
- Lower the dumbbells back to shoulder height as you inhale.
- Maintain controlled and gentle movements.
- Repeat 8 to 15 presses.
- Perform 2 to 5 sets of this exercise.

If you find this exercise too difficult to do you can start off with an even lighter dumbbell to reduce the resistance.

You could also try performing the exercise while seated on a sturdy chair or a bench to provide you with better stability.

You could use one dumbbell at a time if doing both at one time feels too challenging for you.

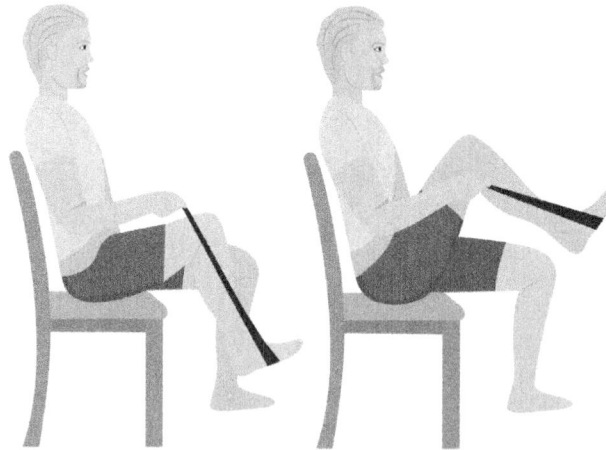

- Using a resistance band, sit on a chair and loop the resistance band under your foot.
- Engage your core muscles as you begin belly breathing pulling your belly button toward your spine.
- Push through your heels and extend your leg.
- You should feel the pull in your calves and hamstrings as you pull the resistance bands with the bottom of your feet.
- Extend your knees without locking them.
- Hold this position for a few seconds as you feel the contractions in your quadriceps.
- Slowly, begin to bend your knees to release the stretch of the resistance band.
- Your movements must be controlled and at a gentle pace.
- Repeat 8 to 15 presses.
- Perform 2 to 5 sets.

If this exercise is too difficult, you can modify it by using a lower resistance level band.

You could also try performing the exercise with a partial range of motion.

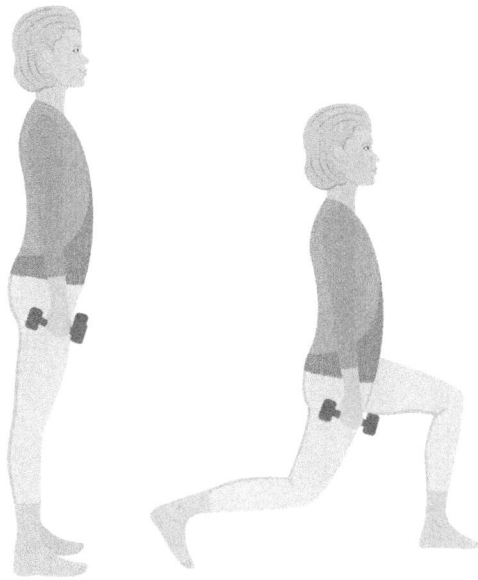

- You will need to use dumbbells or a household weight you can hold onto. Begin by keeping your back straight, your shoulders relaxed, and your core engaged, as you practice deep breathing.
- Take one step forward with your right foot.
- Your knee should be directly above your right ankle.
- Gently begin to lower your body by bending both knees.
- Your left knee should hover just above the ground.
- Your back knee should be a few inches from the floor creating a 90-degree angle with your right knee.
- Ensure that your upper body is upright with your chest up and pointing forward.
- Hold this position for a few seconds before returning to the start position.
- Repeat the lunges following the movements on the other leg, stepping forward with your left foot.
- Continue alternating legs 10 to 15 times.
- Perform 2 to 5 sets.

If it's too difficult to do this exercise, you can start off with lighter dumbbells to reduce the resistance.

You can perform a reverse lunge as you step backward instead of forward, which can be less challenging for your balance.

You could also use a chair or wall for balance and support if needed.

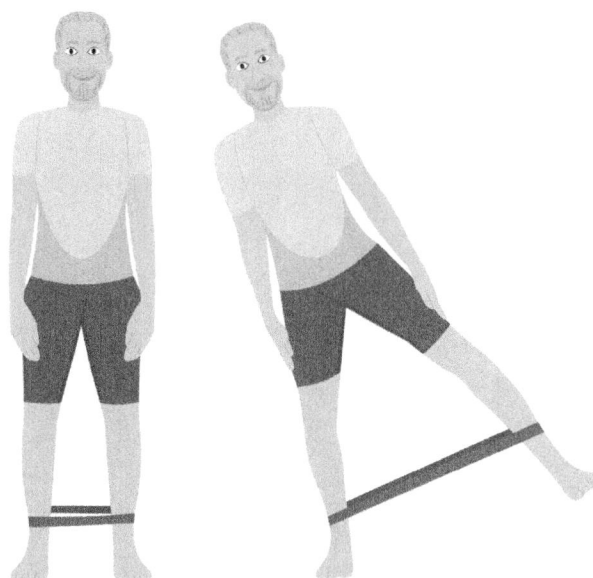

- You are going to need a resistance band for this exercise.
- Start by attaching the band and securing it around your ankles.
- You should stand with your feet hip-width apart and the resistance band should be hooked around both of your ankles.
- Keep your back straight, your shoulders relaxed, and your core engaged as you take deep breaths.
- You can hold onto a chair or a wall for support if needed.
- The resistance band will provide tension as you slowly begin to lift one leg out to the side as far as you comfortably can.
- Your toes should continue pointing forward and you should maintain control throughout the movement.
- Hold the lifted leg position for a few seconds as you feel their engagement in your hip abductor muscles.
- Lower your leg back to the starting position. Repeat this movement with your other leg.
- Continue alternating for 10 to 15 repetitions on each leg.
- Perform 2 to 5 sets.

If it's too difficult for you to do, you can choose a resistance band with less tension.

You can perform this exercise with a smaller range of motion instead of going as far as you can.

You could also hold onto a chair or wall for added support if you feel that standing on one leg is too difficult at the moment.

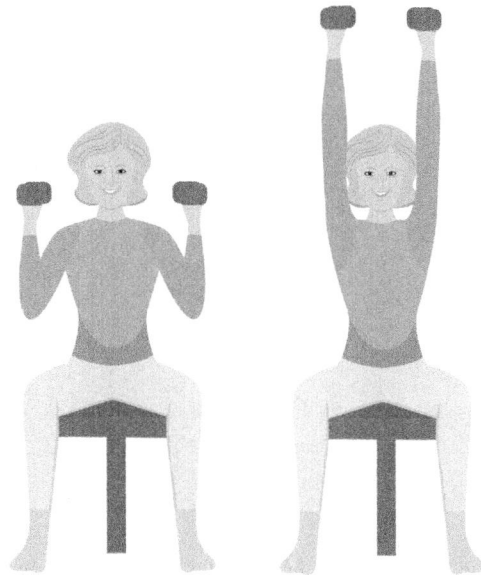

- You are going to need a chair or bench with a backrest and sturdy feet on the ground with two dumbbells for this exercise.
- Begin by sitting down while holding a dumbbell in each hand at shoulder height with your palms facing your shoulders.
- Your elbows should be bent at a 90-degree angle.
- Your back should be straight, shoulders relaxed, and core engaged as you take deep breaths.
- Begin by pushing the dumbbells upward until your arms are fully extended overhead while exhaling.
- Your wrists should be straight and you should avoid locking your elbows.
- Hold this position for a few seconds as you focus on your shoulder muscles.
- Slowly begin to lower the dumbbells back to shoulder height while inhaling.
- Your pace should be controlled throughout the entire exercise.
- Repeat 10 to 15 repetitions of this exercise.
- Perform 2 to 3 sets.

If the exercise is too difficult for you, you can start with lighter dumbbells so that you reduce the resistance.

You can also perform the exercise with one dumbbell at a time.

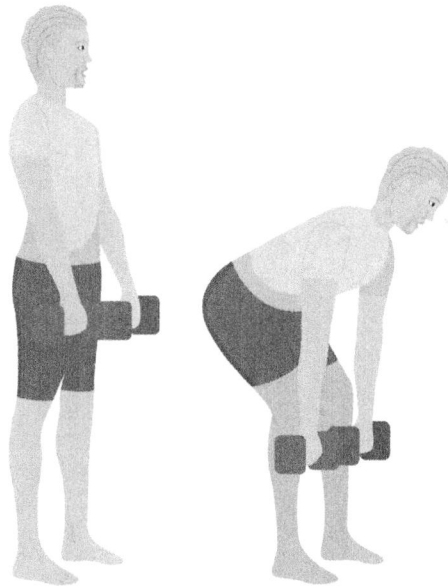

- You will need to have a dumbbell or kettlebell for both of your hands when performing this exercise.
- Begin by standing with your feet hip-width apart, holding a dumbbell or kettlebell in each hand in front of your thighs.
- Keep your back straight, your shoulders relaxed, and your core engaged as you take deep breaths.
- Bend your knees slightly to create a soft bend but maintain a strong but not locked position.
- Hinge at your hips, pushing your buttocks backward and lowering your chest toward the ground.
- Keep the dumbbells close to your legs as you lower them.
- They should remain in contact with your thighs.
- Lower the weights until you feel a stretch in your hamstrings or until they are just below your knees.
- Your back should be straight throughout this movement.
- Pause for a few seconds at the bottom of the deadlift.
- Engage your glutes and hamstrings to return to the standing position.
- Your weights should be close to your legs as you stand up.
- Repeat 8 to 10 repetitions of this exercise.
- Perform 2 to 5 sets.

If it's too difficult to do these lifts, you can modify them by starting with lighter dumbbells or kettlebells.

You could also perform the exercise using a chair behind you to act as a guide for your range of motion.

You could use a mirror or have a trainer check your form and ensure that you are maintaining a straight back throughout the movements.

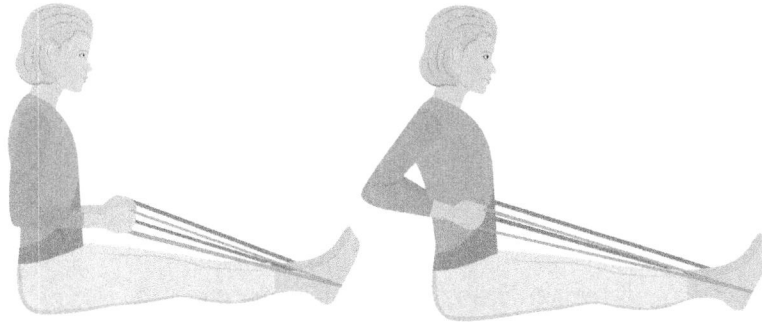

- For this exercise you can do them using resistance bands.
- First, sit down on a mat.
- Place the resistance band around your feet.
- Try to pull the bands with both arms.
- Your elbows should move as back as they can comfortably.
- After you have held the position for a few seconds, slowly extend your arms to return to the starting position.
- Your pace should be controlled.
- Repeat this exercise 8 to 15 times.
- Perform 2 to 5 sets.

If the exercise is too difficult, you can start with a lower-intensity resistance band.

You can adjust your range of motion cooling only as far as your back instead of moving your elbows behind your back. This reduces the effort needed.

49

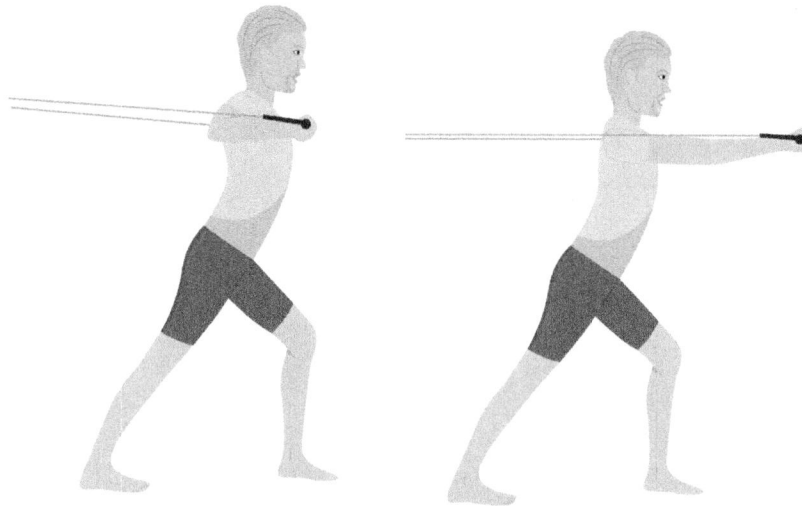

- You will need a resistance band for this exercise.
- Begin by securing the resistance band to a steady anchor point or using a door attachment.
- You should stand with your feet shoulder-width apart as you face away from the anchor point.
- Your hand should hold the ends of the resistance band, each hand palm facing down.
- Gently take a step forward with one foot to create tension in the resistance band.
- Your back should be kept straight, your shoulders relaxed, and your core engaged with deep breathing.
- Start with using your hands, elbows bent at a 90-degree angle as you push them forward, extending them fully while exhaling.
- Keep your movement controlled.
- Hold this position for a few seconds as you feel the concentration in your chest muscles.
- Slowly, return your hands to chest level while inhaling.
- Maintaining control as you continue with this exercise, repeat 10 to 15 times.
- Perform 2 to 5 sets.

To make this exercise easier you can choose a resistance band with low tension. You could also do this in a seated position for better stability and support.

You can choose to do it with a shorter range of motion as you don't fully extend your arms.

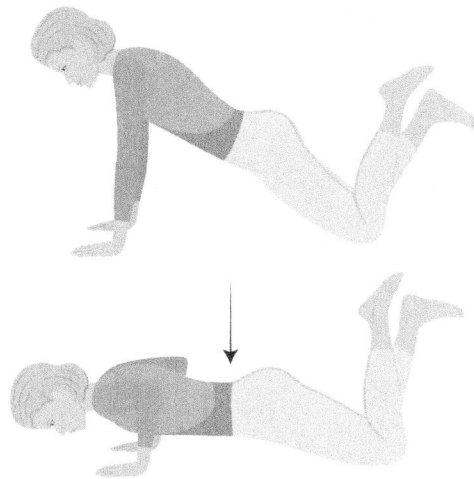

- You will need to first begin to get into a tabletop position with your hands and knees on a mat or soft surface.
- Your hands should be placed slightly wider than shoulder-width apart
- Your palms must be flat on the ground and your fingers pointing forward.
- Your knees should be placed together, bent at 90-degree angles.
- Engage your core muscles as you pull your belly button towards your spine with deep breathing.
- Lower your upper body toward the ground by bending your elbows while keeping your back straight.
- Go as low as you can comfortably without touching your chest to the ground.
- Pause for a moment at the bottom of the push-up before pushing through your palms to straighten them and return to the starting position.
- Your pace should be controlled and gentle throughout the exercise.
- Do not lock your elbows.
- Repeat this exercise 8 to 15 times.
- Perform 2 to 3 sets.

If this exercise is too difficult for you, you can adjust the width of your knees to provide more stability and support.

You could use a cushion or pad under your knees to reduce any discomfort.

You could also start with a shallow range of motion.

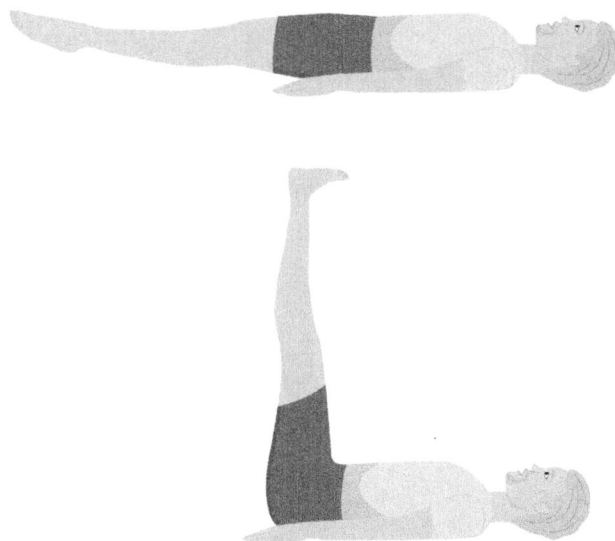

- Begin by lying down on a mat.
- Your body should be aligned from your feet to your neck, and head.
- Your hands should be placed on your sides, palms facing down.
- Engage your core muscles, pulling your belly button toward your spine with deep breathing.
- Slowly lift your legs off the ground, extending them straight in front of you.
- Increase the height of your lifted legs until they form a 45-degree angle with the ground.
- Hold this position for a few seconds before lowering your legs back down to the ground.
- Repeat this exercise 8 to 15 times.
- Perform 2 to 5 sets.

If this exercise is too difficult for you to hold your position, you can perform it with a smaller range of motion where you lift your leg only a few inches off the ground.

You can also do this using one leg at a time.

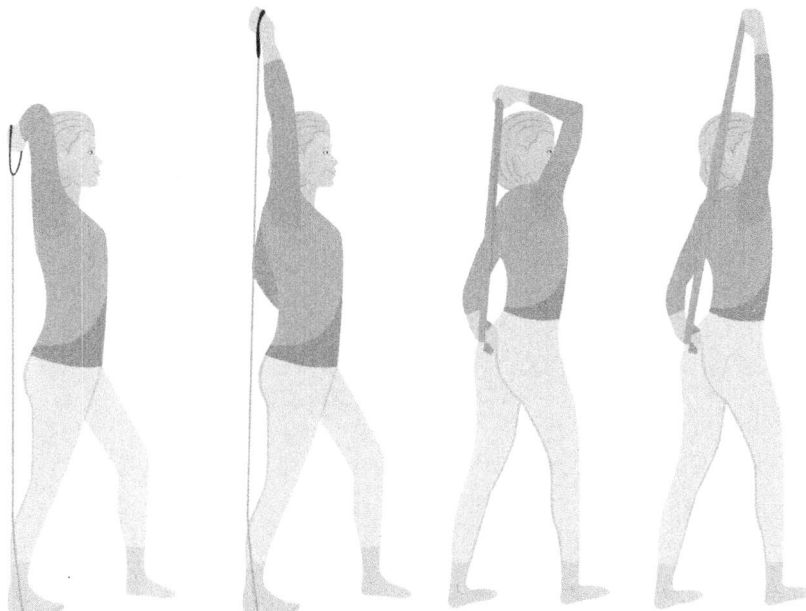

- You will need a resistance band for this exercise.
- Begin by securing the resistance bands to a sturdy anchor behind you, for example, you could place it under your foot or use one hand to hold it behind your back.
- Using your other hand, take the other end of the resistance band and hold it with a firm grip.
- Keeping your back straight, your shoulders relaxed and the core engaged with deep breathing, begin to move by lifting one arm in front of you.
- Bend the arm at a 90-degree angle.
- Your elbow should be close to your side and your hand must be at shoulder level.
- Continue pulling the band until you reach overhead.
- Your elbow should be fully extended as you straighten your arm.
- Your arm holding the band behind you should be stationary during this movement.
- If you are using your foot to hold down the resistance band, ensure that both your arms are grasping onto the resistance band overhead.
- Hold the extended position for a few seconds as you feel the contraction in your triceps muscle.
- Slowly return your hand to the starting position while inhaling.
- Your pace should be controlled.
- Repeat this exercise 8 to 15 times.

- If you use one hand to perform the exercise, repeat the same number of repetitions on the other.
- Perform 2 to 5 sets.

If this is too difficult for you to do, you can choose a resistance band with lower tension.

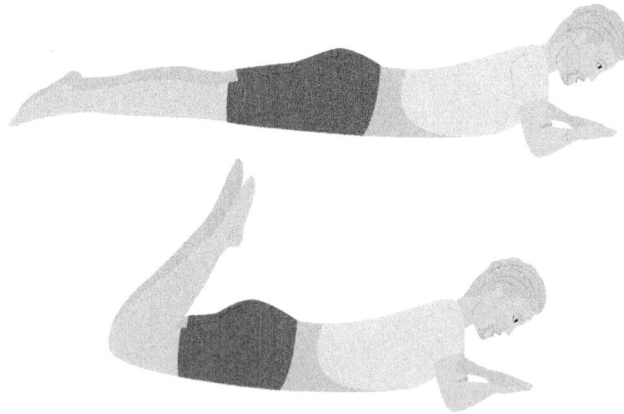

- Begin by lying down on your front on a soft padded material.
- Keep your back straight, your shoulders relaxed, and your core engaged as you breathe deeply.
- Start by flexing your knees, curling your lower legs toward your buttocks while exhaling.
- Your upper legs and upper body must be stationary during the movement.
- Hold the curved position for a moment, feeling the contraction in your hamstring muscles.
- Slowly extend your legs, returning to the starting position.
- Your movements should be gentle and controlled.
- Repeat the movements 8 to 15 times.
- Perform 2 to 5 sets.

To modify this exercise and make it easier, you should use a cushion or pad on the floor under your legs for some added comfort.

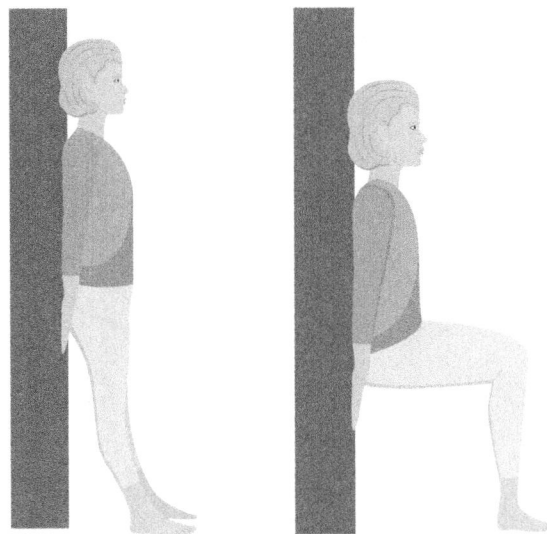

- Begin by finding a sturdy and clear wall space.
- You should stand with your back against the wall.
- Your feet must be shoulder-width apart.
- Your feet must be flat on the ground and your toes should be pointing slightly outward.
- Gently, begin to slide your back down while bending your knees until they are at a 90-degree angle.
- It should look as though you are sitting in an imaginary chair.
- Your knees must be directly above your ankles.
- Your thighs must be parallel to the ground.
- Your back should be against the wall.
- Your shoulders and head must be relaxed.
- As you stay in this position, your core muscles must be engaged as you practice deep breathing.
- This position should be held for as long as you can, aiming for a specific time duration ranging between 20 to 30 seconds.
- Maintain proper form and breathing throughout this exercise.
- To exit this position gently slide back after while pushing through the balls of your feet as you straighten your legs.
- Perform 2 to 5 sets of this exercise.

If this exercise is too difficult for you to perform, you can do a shallow wall sit where you bend your knees less than 90°.

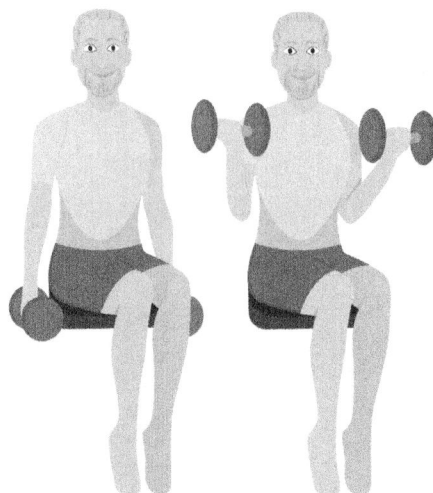

- You will need a chair or sturdy bench and dumbbells to perform this exercise.
- Begin by sitting down with your back straight and feet flat on the ground.
- Your knees must be at a 90-degree angle.
- Hold a dumbbell in each hand as you allow your arms to hang loosely by your side.
- Your palms should be facing your legs.
- Your back must be straight, your shoulders relaxed, and your core engaged as you begin deep breathing.
- Begin by flexing your elbow, and lifting the dumbbells towards your shoulders while exhaling.
- Ensure that your upper arms are stationary and close to your body during these movements.
- Squeeze your biceps at the top of the curl as you hold the position for a few seconds.
- Feel the contraction in your biceps before gently lowering the dumbbells back down to the starting position as you breathe in.
- Your pace should be controlled.
- Repeat 10 to 15 curls.
- Perform 2 to 3 sets of this exercise.

If this exercise is too difficult for you to do, you can modify it by starting with lighter dumbbells to reduce the resistance.

You can also perform the exercise one arm at a time.

You could use a chair with armrests for added support and stability.

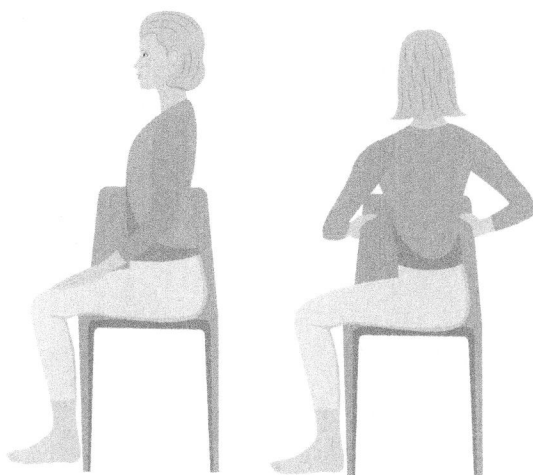

- To begin, you will need a sturdy chair.
- Sit down with your back straight and feet flat on the ground.
- Your knees must be at a 90-degree angle.
- Keep your core engaged as you practice deep breathing, feeling as though you are pulling your belly button towards your spine.
- Keep your hands on your hips or hold onto the sides of the chair for stability.
- You can start your movements by rotating your upper body to the right.
- Your hips and lower body must still be facing forward.
- Twist as far as you can comfortably without straining any of your muscles.
- Hold this position for a few seconds as you feel the stretch or engagement in your oblique muscles
- Slowly return to the starting position as you face forward.
- Repeat this twist rotating your upper body to the left this time.
- Hold this position for a few seconds before returning to the start position.
- Continue alternating twists from the left to the right 8 to 15 times.
- Perform 2 to 3 sets of the exercise.

If you feel that this exercise is too difficult for you to do you must begin with smaller twists so that you aren't going too far on each side.

You could also use the chair's backrest for some added stability.

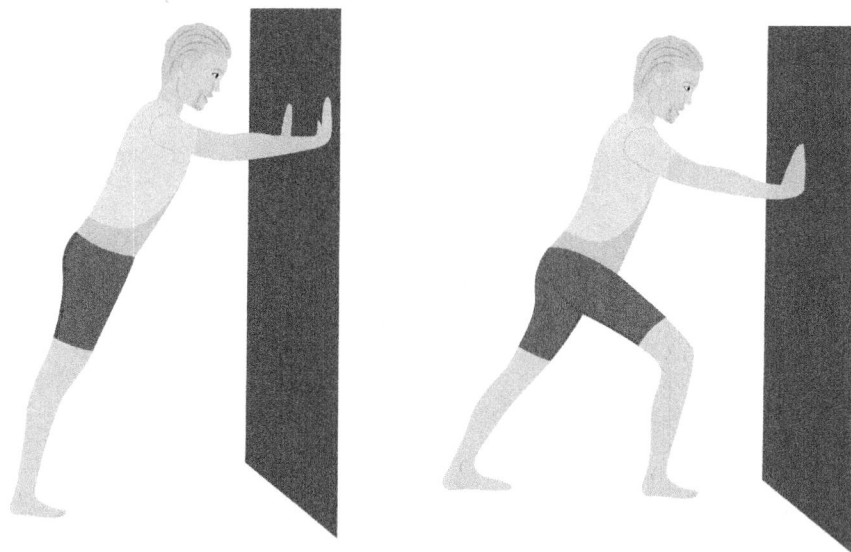

- You will need to do this exercise next to a wall.
- Begin by standing facing the clear wall space.
- Your feet should be hip-width apart and a comfortable distance away from the wall.
- Place your hands against the wall.
- Your arms should be at shoulder height and straight.
- Take a step back with your right foot as you keep both heels flat on the ground.
- Then lift your left knee slightly while keeping your right leg straight. This should create a stretch in your right calf.
- Your right toes must be pointing directly forward.
- Your back should be straight and your core engaged as you breathe deeply.
- Hold this position for 15 to 30 seconds.
- Release the stretch and return to a neutral position
- Repeat the movements with your left foot as you stretch your left calf.
- Hold this position again for 15 to 30 seconds.
- Repeat alternating movements 10 to 15 times on each leg.
- Perform 2 to 5 sets of this exercise.

To make it easier, use a higher will surface to reduce the intensity.

You could also do this while seated with your legs extended as you gently flex and point your toes to stretch out your calves.

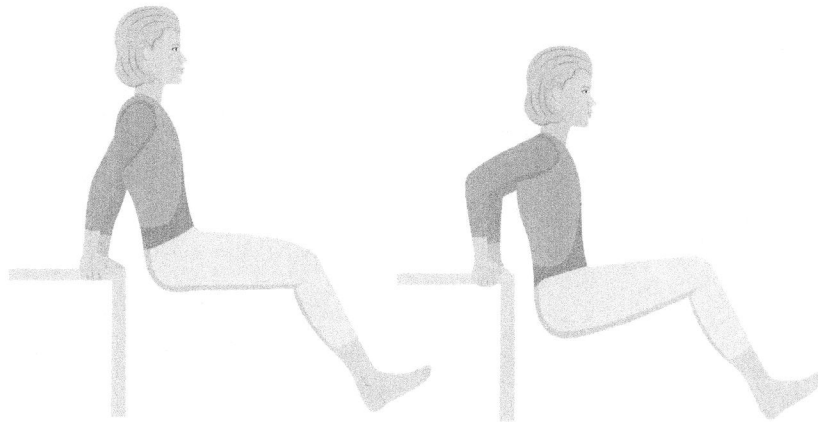

- To do this exercise you need a sturdy chair.
- You will begin by placing the chair with its back against the wall.
- Stand in front of the chair, facing away with your feet hip-width apart.
- Hold on to the chair with your hands, palms facing downward and fingers scraping the front edge.
- Move your feet forward a few steps, extending your legs so that your knees are slightly bent.
- Keep your back straight, your shoulders relaxed, and your core engaged.
- Start by lowering your body toward the ground by bending your elbows.
- Lower your body until your elbows are bent at about a 90-degree angle or slightly less.
- Hold this position for a few seconds as you feel the engagement in your tricep muscles.
- Push through your palms gently to straighten your arms and return to the starting position.
- Your pace should be controlled throughout the exercise.
- Repeat these movements 8 to 15 times.
- Perform 2 to 3 sets.

If this exercise is too difficult for you to do, you can modify it by performing the exercise with your knees more bent to reduce the intensity.

You could also use a chair with armrests for added support and stability.

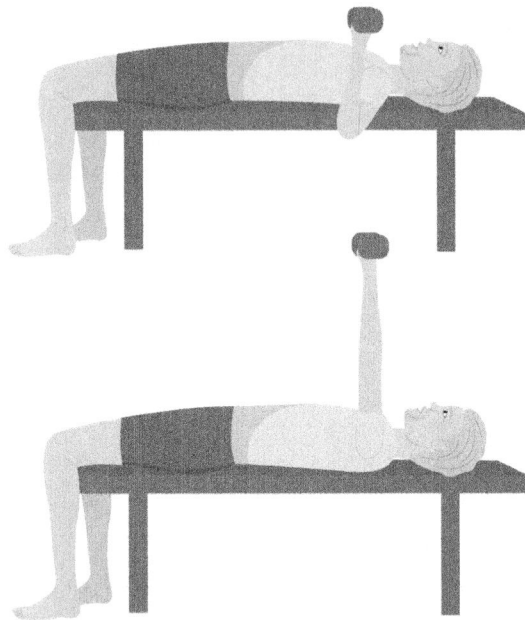

- For this exercise, you will need a sturdy long bench or coffee table that can support your weight.
- Begin by lying down on the bench, your feet flat on the ground and your knees bent at a 90-degree angle.
- Hold a dumbbell in each hand and position them at chest level with your palms facing forward.
- Your back must be against the bench, your shoulders relaxed, and your core engaged.
- Slowly start the exercise by lifting the dumbbells upward until your arms fully extend facing up.
- Avoid knocking your elbows.
- Hold this position for 3 seconds as you focus on your chest muscles.
- Slowly lower the dumbbells back to the start position while inhaling.
- Your pace should be controlled throughout this exercise.
- Repeat these movements 10 to 15 times.
- Perform 2 to 3 sets of this exercise.

If these exercises are too difficult for you to do, you can modify them by starting with lighter dumbbells to reduce the resistance.

You could also perform the exercise with one dumbbell at a time if using both hands feels too challenging.

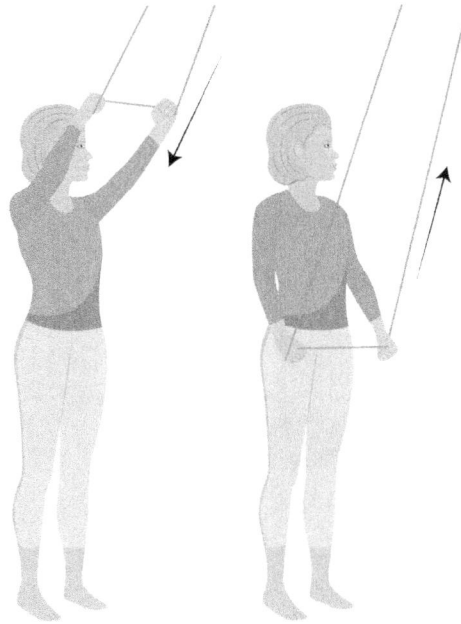

- To do this exercise, you will need a resistance band and a sturdy anchor point that is above you.
- Attach the resistance band above you.
- Stand facing the anchor point.
- Hold the end of the resistance bands with both hands facing forward.
- Your back, legs, and head should be aligned.
- Your shoulders should be relaxed.
- Your core must be engaged as you begin deep breathing.
- Pull the band down towards your chest as you squeeze your shoulder blades together.
- Slowly, begin to return your hands to the starting position after holding the stretch for 15 to 30 seconds.
- Repeat 5 to 10 times.
- Perform 2 to 5 sets of this exercise.

If the exercise is too difficult for you, you can choose a resistance band with less tension.

You could also perform the exercise seated for better stability.

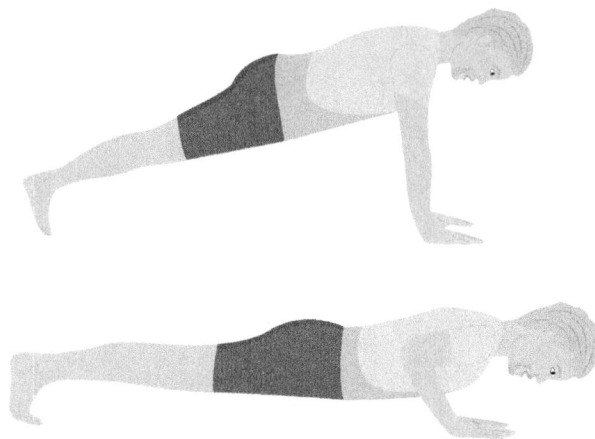

- Begin by getting down into a plank position, your hands placed on the floor slightly wider than shoulder-width apart.
- Your legs should be extended straight behind you with your toes on the ground.
- Your body must be in a straight line from your head to your heels as you begin engaging your core muscles with deep breathing.
- Your wrists must be aligned with your shoulders and your fingers should be pointing forward.
- Lower your body toward the ground by bending your elbows while keeping them as close as possible to your sides.
- Continue moving lower until your chest is just a few inches above the ground, or as far as your body will allow you to do this comfortably.
- Remember to maintain a straight line from your head to your heels throughout the movement.
- Your back should not hunch over.
- Stay in the lower position for a few seconds before pushing through your palms to straighten your arms and return to the starting position while breathing out.
- Keep your core engaged to prevent yourself from sagging.
- Repeat this exercise 8 to 15 times.
- Perform 2 to 3 sets of this exercise.

If it's too difficult for you to perform this exercise, you can do it while facing the wall.

You could also perform the movements as you keep your knees on the ground but still maintain your body in a straight line.

You could also use a higher surface like a sturdy countertop, to reduce the angle and make it easier for you.

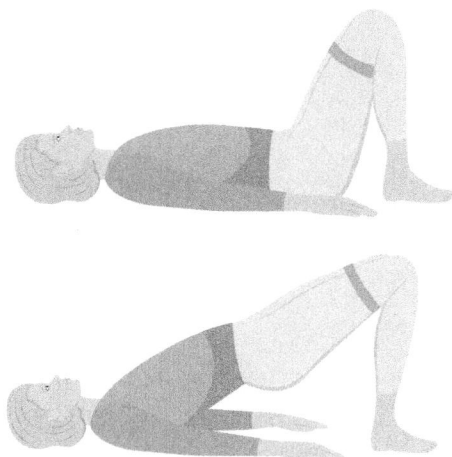

- Begin to exercise while lying down on your back.
- You should use a carpet or yoga mat.
- Bend your knees and place your feet flat on the ground, hip-width apart.
- Your arms should be extended along your sides with your palms facing down for stability.
- Your core muscles should be engaged as you pull your belly button toward your spine.
- Begin the exercise by pushing through your heels and lifting your hips upward, toward the ceiling.
- While in midair, squeeze your glutes.
- Ensure that your body forms a straight line from your shoulders to your legs.
- Hold this position for a few seconds as you feel the contraction in your gluteal muscles.
- Gently, lower your hips back down to the ground while inhaling but don't let them touch the ground completely.
- Repeat this exercise 8 to 15 times holding the position for 10 seconds at a time.
- Perform 2 to 3 sets of this exercise.

If you would like to modify this exercise to make it easier, you could also use a cushion or pad under your shoulder for some added support and comfort.

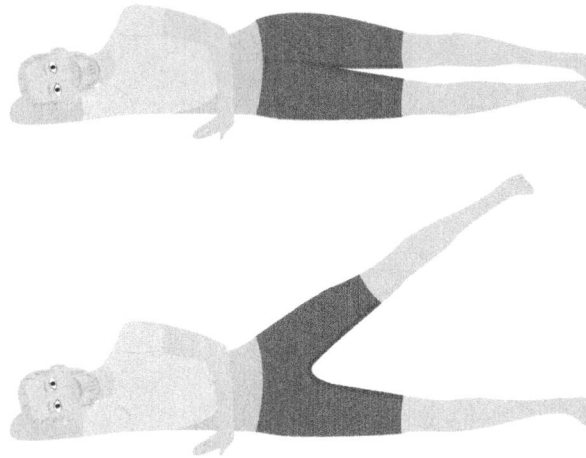

- You will need to lie down on your side on a mat or on a carpet on the floor.
- Your legs should be extended straight.
- Position your lower arm under your head for support and use your upper arm to stabilize your upper body by placing your hand flat on the ground in front of you.
- Your top leg should be attached directly on top of the bottom leg.
- Engage your core muscles as you practice deep breathing, pulling your belly button toward your spine.
- Start by lifting your top leg as high as comfortably possible while exhaling.
- Your leg should be straight and your toes pointing forward.
- Hold the position of your leg for a moment as you feel the engagement in your outer thigh muscles.
- Lower your back down to the starting position as you breathe in.
- Repeat this exercise 8 to 15 times on one side before switching around and performing the same number of repetitions on the other leg.
- Perform 2 to 5 sets of this exercise.

If it's too difficult for you to perform this exercise, you can do the lift with a slight bend in your bottom leg to reduce the intensity.

You could also use a cushion or pad under your lower hip to add comfort and support.

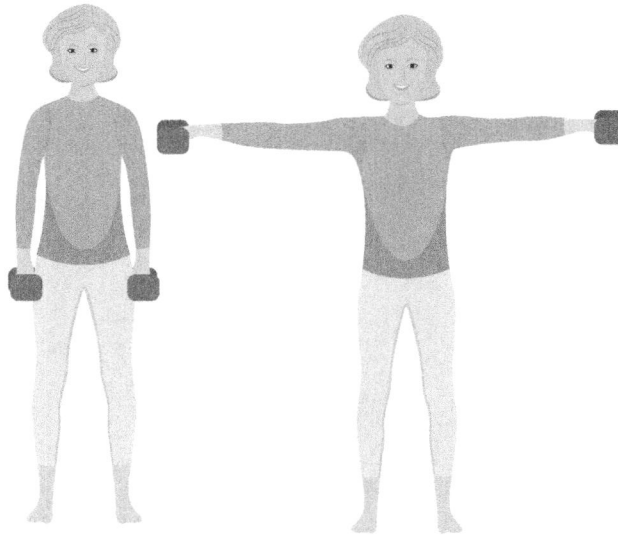

- You will need dumbbells to perform this exercise.
- Begin by standing with your feet hip-width apart.
- Hold a dumbbell in each hand.
- With your palms facing your body, keep your back straight, shoulders relaxed, and core engaged.
- Try to maintain a slight bend in your elbows throughout this exercise.
- Start by lifting up the dumbbells sideways until your arms are parallel to the ground.
- This movement should be done as you breathe out.
- Keep your arms extended and your wrists neutral, avoid bending them.
- Also avoids sagging your body during the movement.
- Remember to use controlled motion.
- Hold the position for 2 to 3 seconds before slowly lowering the dumbbells back to your sides as you breathe in.
- Repeat this exercise 8 to 15 times.
- Perform 2 to 3 sets.

If it's too difficult for you to do this exercise, you can modify it by using lighter dumbbells to reduce the resistance.

You can also do the exercise one arm at a time.

Another alternative is to use a chair or bench for added support and stability.

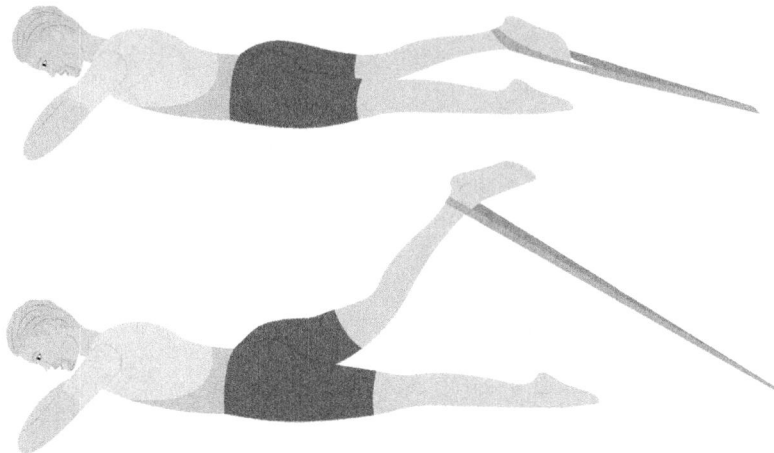

- Begin by securing a resistance band to a sturdy anchor point or using a door attachment.
- Lie face down on an exercise mat or the floor with your legs fully extended.
- Loop the resistance band around your ankle and hold onto the anchor end with your hands.
- Position your arms under your chest for support, with your palms facing down.
- Engage your core muscles by pulling your belly button toward your spine.
- Start the exercise by bending your knee and curling your leg toward your buttocks while exhaling.
- Keep your foot flexed and your toes pointing upward throughout the movement.
- Squeeze your glutes at the top of the curl.
- Hold the curled position for a moment, feeling the contraction in your hamstring muscles.
- Slowly extend your leg back to the starting position while inhaling.
- Maintain a controlled pace throughout the exercise.
- Repeat the exercise 8 to 15 times on each leg.
- Perform 2 to 5 sets.

To make the exercise easier you can modify it by using a lighter resistance band to reduce the tension.

You could also perform the exercise with a smaller range of motion.

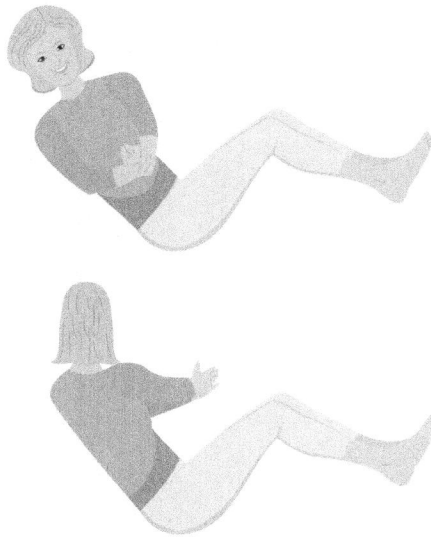

- Begin by sitting on an exercise mat or the floor with your knees bent and your feet flat on the ground.
- Lean back slightly, creating a V-shape with your torso and thighs.
- Keep your back straight, shoulders relaxed, and core engaged.
- Extend your arms straight in front of you, palms together.
- Start the exercise by twisting your torso to the right side while exhaling.
- Keep your arms extended as you rotate, bringing your hands to the outside of your right hip.
- Hold the twisted position for a moment, feeling the engagement in your oblique muscles.
- Return to the center, facing forward while inhaling.
- Repeat the twist, this time rotating your torso to the left side.
- Hold the left twist for a moment before returning to the center.
- Continue alternating twists to the right and left 10 to 15 times on each side.
- Perform 2 to 4 sets.

To make this exercise easier, you can perform it with your heels resting on the ground for added stability.

You could also hold on to a light dumbbell or water bottle with both your hands to add balance and support.

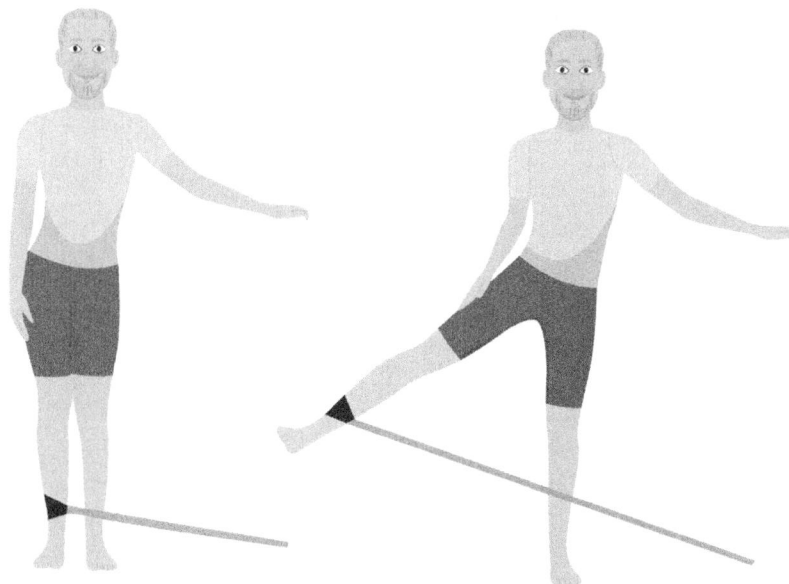

- Begin by securing a resistance band around your ankles or above your knees.
- Stand with your feet hip-width apart and your toes pointing forward.
- Keep your back straight, shoulders relaxed, and core engaged.
- Place your hands on your hips or hold onto a stable surface for support.
- Start the exercise by lifting your right leg out to the side as far as comfortably possible while exhaling.
- Keep your leg straight but not locked and maintain tension on the resistance band.
- Hold the raised position for a moment, feeling the engagement in your hip abductors (outer hip muscles).
- Lower your right leg back down to the starting position while inhaling.
- Repeat the exercise 10 to 12 times on your right leg.
- Switch to your left leg and perform the same number of repetitions.
- Perform 2 to 5 sets.

If this exercise is too difficult for you, you can use a lighter resistance band to reduce the tension.

You could also perform it with a much smaller range of motion.

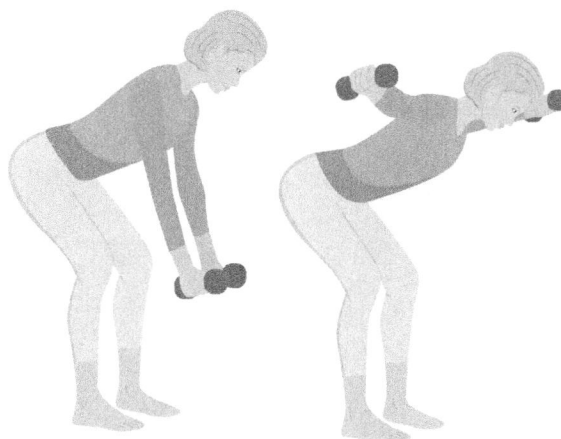

- Begin by standing with your feet hip-width apart, holding a dumbbell in each hand by your sides, palms facing your thighs.
- Keep your back straight, shoulders relaxed, and core engaged.
- Maintain a slight bend in your knees throughout the exercise.
- Start the exercise by hinging at your hips and bending forward at a 45-degree angle.
- Keep your arms fully extended toward the ground, perpendicular to your torso.
- Begin the movement by raising both dumbbells out to the sides while exhaling.
- Keep your elbows slightly bent during the motion and focus on using your rear shoulder muscles.
- Squeeze your shoulder blades together at the top of the fly.
- Hold the raised position for a moment, feeling the contraction in your rear shoulders.
- Slowly lower the dumbbells back to your sides while inhaling.
- Maintain a controlled pace throughout the exercise.
- Repeat the exercise 8 to 10 times.
- Perform 2 to 3 sets.

To make this exercise easier, you can start with lighter dumbbells.

You could also perform the exercise one arm at a time. L

Instead of standing you can use a chair or bench for some added support and stability.

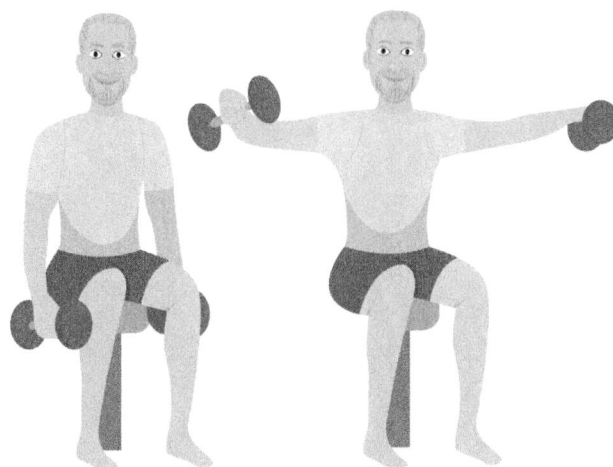

- Begin by sitting on a sturdy chair or bench with your back straight, feet flat on the ground, and knees at a 90-degree angle.
- Hold a dumbbell in each hand by your sides, palms facing your thighs.
- Keep your back against the chair's backrest, shoulders relaxed, and core engaged.
- Maintain a slight bend in your elbows throughout the exercise.
- Begin the exercise by lifting both dumbbells out to the sides until they are at shoulder level or slightly below while exhaling.
- Keep your arms extended and your wrists neutral.
- Avoid swinging your body during the movement; use controlled motion.
- Hold the raised position for a moment, feeling the engagement in your shoulder muscles.
- Slowly lower the dumbbells back to your sides while inhaling.
- Maintain a controlled pace throughout the exercise.
- Repeat the exercise 8 to 15 times.
- Perform 2 to 4 sets.

To decrease the difficulty level you can start with lighter dumbbells to reduce the resistance.

You could also perform the exercise one arm at a time.

You could also sit on a chair with back support to aid with your stability.

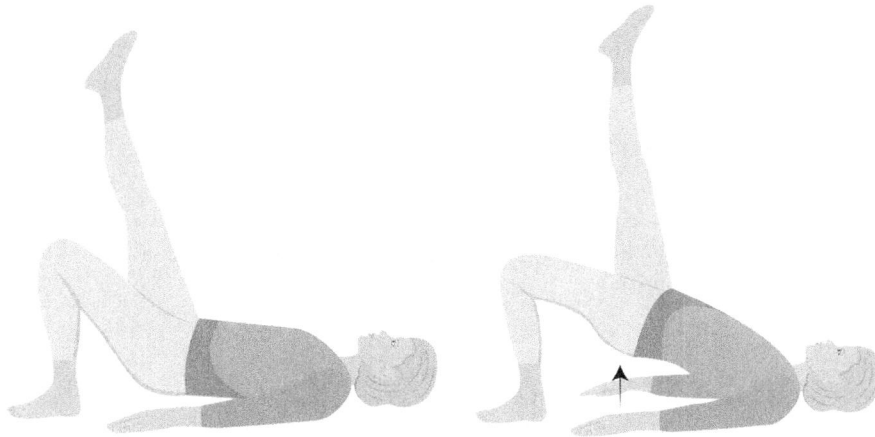

- Begin by lying on your back on an exercise mat or the floor with your knees bent and feet flat on the ground, hip-width apart.
- Place your arms by your sides with your palms facing down.
- Engage your core muscles by pulling your belly button toward your spine.
- Start the exercise by pressing through your heels and lifting your hips upward toward the ceiling while exhaling.
- Squeeze your glutes at the top of the bridge.
- Maintain the bridge position while you raise one leg straight up toward the ceiling.
- Keep your raised leg straight but not locked and your toes pointed.
- Hold the raised position for a moment, feeling the engagement in your gluteal muscles.
- Lower your raised leg back down to the ground.
- Lower your hips back down to the ground while inhaling.
- Repeat the exercise, this time raising the other leg.
- Continue alternating leg lifts in the bridge position for 8 to 12 times on each leg
- Perform 2 to 4 sets.

To make this exercise easier, you can perform it without raising your hips as high.

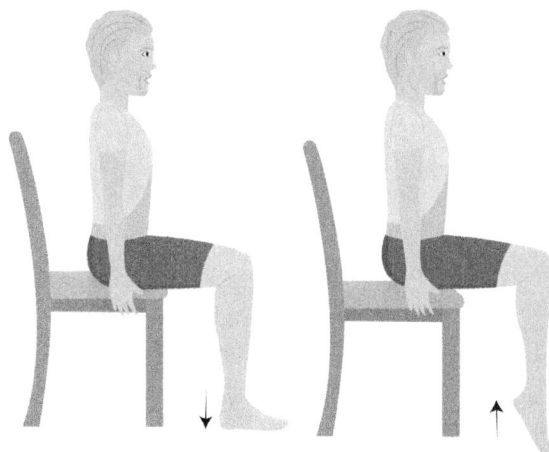

- Begin by sitting on a sturdy chair or bench with your back straight, feet flat on the ground, and knees at a 90-degree angle.
- Place your hands on your thighs or on the sides of the chair for support.
- Position the balls of your feet on the edge of a step or a block, allowing your heels to hang off the edge.
- Keep your back straight, shoulders relaxed, and core engaged.
- Start the exercise by pressing through the balls of your feet and lifting your heels as high as comfortably possible while exhaling.
- Focus on contracting your calf muscles as you raise your heels.
- Hold the raised position for a moment, feeling the engagement in your calf muscles.
- Lower your heels back down below the level of the step or block while inhaling.
- Maintain a controlled pace throughout the exercise.
- Repeat the exercise 8 to 12 times.
- Perform 2 to 3 sets.

To make this exercise easier, you can use a lower step or block to reduce the range of motion.

You could also perform the exercise with both feet together for added stability.

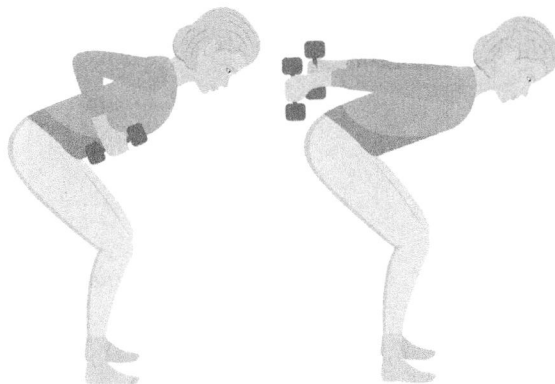

- Begin by standing with your feet hip-width apart, holding a dumbbell in each hand.
- Keep your back straight, shoulders relaxed, and core engaged.
- Hold the dumbbells by your sides, palms facing your body.
- Maintain a slight bend in your knees throughout the exercise.
- Start the exercise by hinging at your hips and bending your upper body forward at about a 45-degree angle.
- Keep your elbows close to your sides, bent at a 90-degree angle.
- Begin the movement by extending your arms straight back behind you while exhaling.
- Fully extend your arms so that they are parallel to the ground, keeping your upper arms still.
- Hold the extended position for a moment, focusing on your tricep muscles.
- Slowly bend your elbows to return the dumbbells to the starting position while inhaling.
- Maintain a controlled pace throughout the exercise.
- Repeat the exercise 8 to 12 times.
- Perform 2 to 4 sets.

To make this exercise easier you can start off with lighter dumbbells.

You could also perform the exercise with one at a time. You could use a chair or a bench for added support and stability as well.

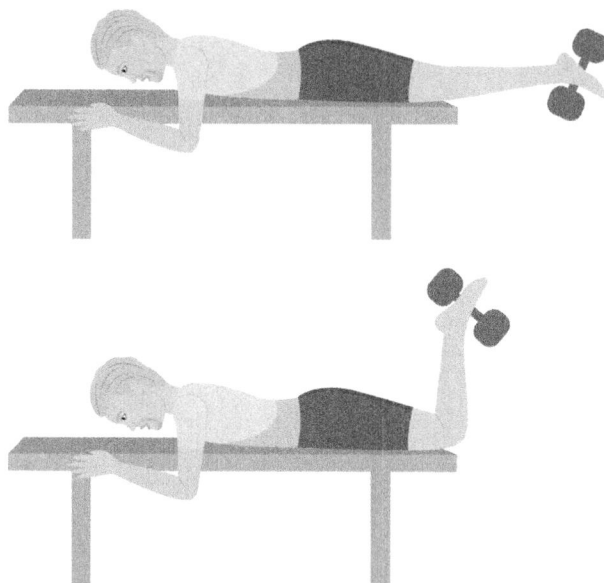

- Begin by lying face down on an exercise mat on the floor, or a bench, with your legs fully extended.
- Place your arms by your sides, palms facing up, or use your hands to support your forehead for comfort.
- Engage your core muscles by pulling your belly button toward your spine.
- Start the exercise by putting a weight between your feet.
- Bend your knees and curl your heels toward your buttocks while exhaling.
- Keep your thighs and hips on the ground throughout the movement.
- Squeeze your hamstring muscles as you curl your heels as close to your buttocks as possible.
- Hold the curled position for a moment, feeling the contraction in your hamstrings.
- Slowly lower your heels back to the starting position while inhaling.
- Maintain a controlled pace throughout the exercise.
- Repeat the exercise 8 to 15 times.
- Perform 2 to 4 sets.

To make this exercise easier you can start with a smaller range of motion.

You could also put a cushion or pad under your hips to offer added comfort and support.

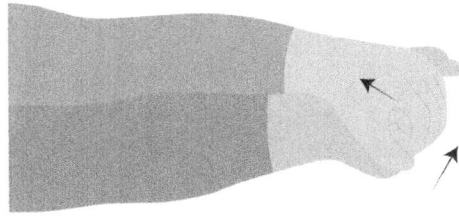

- Begin by sitting or standing in a comfortable position.
- Extend your right arm straight in front of you with your palm facing down.
- Use your left hand to gently grasp your right fingers and apply light pressure to pull them back toward your body.
- You should feel a stretch in your forearm and along the underside of your wrist.
- Hold the stretch for 15 to 30 seconds while breathing deeply and evenly.
- Release your right hand and shake out your wrist and fingers to release tension.
- Repeat the stretch on the left arm, extending it straight in front of you with the palm facing down and using your right hand to gently pull back on the fingers.
- Hold the stretch for 15 to 30 seconds.
- Release and shake out your wrist and fingers again.
- Repeat on your other arm.
- Perform 2 to 4 sets.

To make this easier, you can perform the stretch with your arms bent at a 90-degree angle.

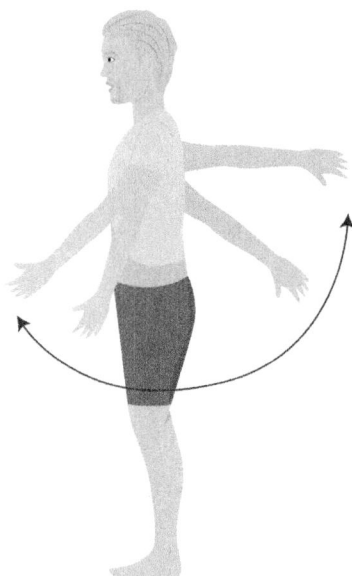

- Begin by standing up straight with your feet shoulder-width apart.
- Position your arms at your sides, with your palms facing inward.
- Start the exercise by gently swinging your arms forward and backward in a controlled and fluid motion.
- As you swing your arms forward, cross them in front of your body, one over the other.
- As you swing your arms backward, open them wide, moving them away from each other.
- Keep your movements relaxed and smooth, and focus on the natural swinging motion.
- Continue swinging your arms for about 30 seconds to 1 minute.
- Perform 2 to 4 sets.

You can vary the speed of your arm swings depending on your comfort level and mobility.

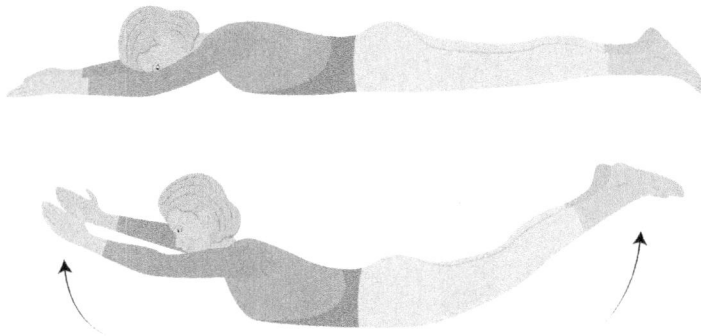

- Begin by lying face down on an exercise mat or the floor with your legs fully extended and your arms stretched out overhead.
- Keep your palms facing down and your toes pointing toward the floor.
- Engage your core muscles by pulling your belly button toward your spine.
- Start the exercise by simultaneously lifting your arms, chest, and legs off the ground while exhaling.
- Keep your arms and legs straight but not locked.
- Aim to create a flying position, with only your abdomen and pelvis remaining in contact with the ground.
- Hold the raised position for a moment, squeezing your glutes and lower back muscles.
- Lower your arms, chest, and legs back down to the ground while inhaling.
- Maintain a controlled pace throughout the exercise.
- Repeat the exercise 6 to 12 times.
- Perform 2 to 3 sets.

To make this easier you can lift only your upper body off the ground and leave your legs in their start position.

You can also lift up your legs alone instead of simultaneously with your arms and head.

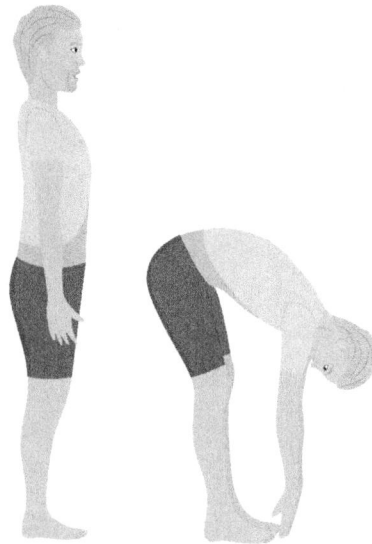

- Begin by standing up straight with your feet together.
- Position your arms at your sides, with your palms facing inward.
- Take a deep breath in.
- As you exhale, bend at your hips and lower your upper body toward the ground.
- Keep your back straight and maintain a slight bend in your knees to prevent overstretching.
- Reach your hands toward your toes or as far down your legs as comfortably possible.
- Hold the stretched position for a moment, feeling the stretch in your hamstrings and lower back.
- Inhale as you slowly return to the starting position, uncurling your upper body.
- Repeat the exercise 8 to 12 times.
- Perform 3 to 5 sets.

To make this easier, you can perform this stretch with a smaller range of motion.

You can also bend your knees slightly.

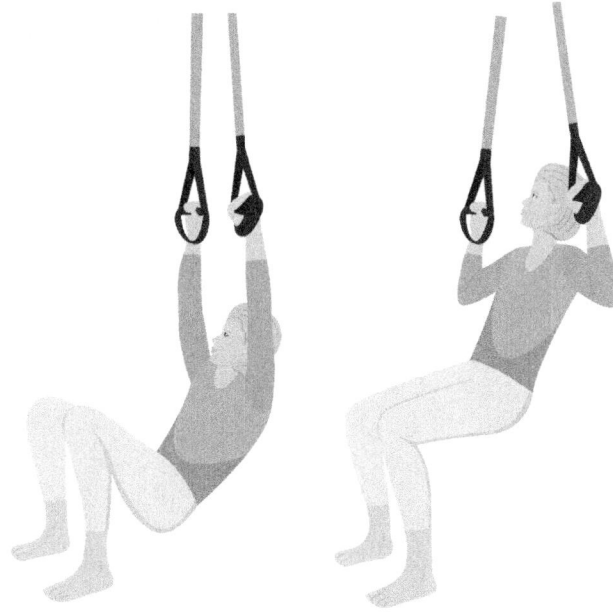

- Use a resistance band that is hooked on something stable above you and can carry your weight.
- Stand facing the bar with your feet hip-width apart.
- Reach up and grasp the bar with both hands, positioning them slightly wider than shoulder-width apart.
- Keep your palms facing forward.
- Bend your knees, your weight moving to your feet and back, so that your arms are fully extended, and you are hanging from the band.
- Allow your body to hang freely, and let your shoulders and arms fully extend.
- Relax your neck, and keep your head in a neutral position.
- Take deep breaths, and focus on feeling the stretch in your lats, which are the broad muscles of your back.
- Hold the stretched position for 15 to 30 seconds, breathing deeply and evenly.
- Perform 2 to 3 sets.
- After the stretch, release the bar and extend your legs up, to return to an upright position.

To modify this, you can use a chair for support.

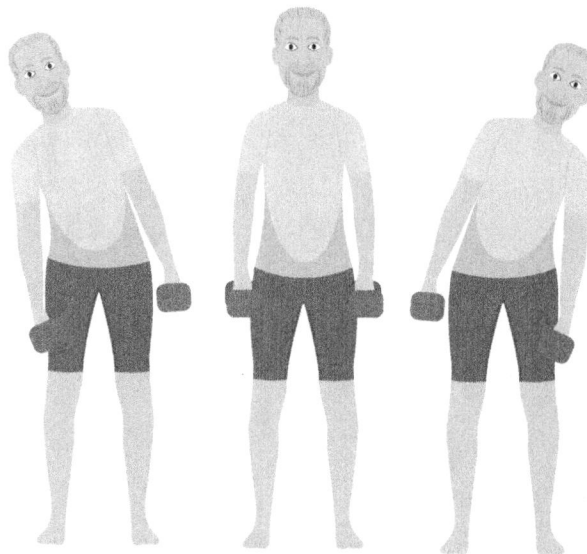

- Begin by standing up straight with your feet shoulder-width apart.
- Position your arms at your sides, with your palms facing inward.
- Take a deep breath in.
- As you exhale, gently bend your upper body to the right side without twisting your torso.
- Keep your feet firmly planted on the ground and maintain a neutral pelvis.
- Stretch your right arm down toward your right knee while sliding your left arm up and over your head, reaching toward the right side.
- Hold the stretched position for a moment, feeling the stretch along your left side.
- Inhale as you slowly return to the upright position.
- Repeat the exercise by bending your upper body to the left side while exhaling.
- Stretch your left arm down toward your left knee and reach your right arm up and over your head toward the left side.
- Hold the stretched position for a moment.
- Continue alternating side bends 6 to 12 times.
- Perform 2 to 3 sets.

To make it easier, you can perform this exercise seated in a chair for added stability.

You could also reduce the range of motion by bending only slightly to each side.

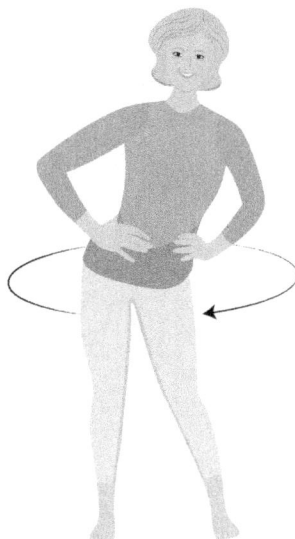

- Begin by standing up straight with your feet hip-width apart.
- Position your hands on your hips or let your arms hang freely at your sides.
- Take a deep breath in.
- As you exhale, start making circular motions with your hips.
- Imagine drawing large circles with your hips, moving them forward, to the right, back, and to the left.
- Keep your upper body relatively still and focus on the movement of your hips.
- Continue making hip circles for about 15 to 30 seconds before stopping.
- Reverse the direction of the circles, moving your hips in the opposite direction, for another 15 to 30 seconds.
- Perform 2 to 3 sets.

To make it simpler, you can perform smaller hip circles if you have limited mobility or feel discomfort during the exercise.

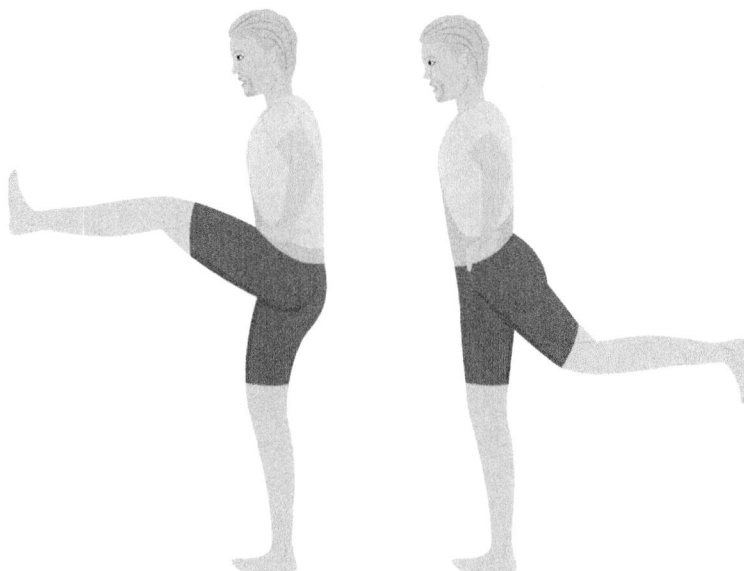

- Begin by standing up straight with your feet close together.
- Position your hands on a stable surface for balance support, such as a wall or a sturdy chair.
- Take a deep breath in, keep your core engaged.
- As you exhale, lift your right leg off the ground a few inches.
- Start swinging your right leg forward and backward in a controlled manner.
- Keep your leg relatively straight but not locked, and maintain a slight bend in your standing knee.
- Swing your leg forward and backward, gradually increasing the range of motion as you warm up.
- Perform the swings for about 15 to 30 seconds.
- Lower your right leg back down to the ground.
- Switch to your left leg and perform leg swings forward and backward for another 15 to 30 seconds.
- Perform 2 to 3 sets.

To make it easier, you can perform smaller leg swings or hold onto a sturdy surface for additional support.

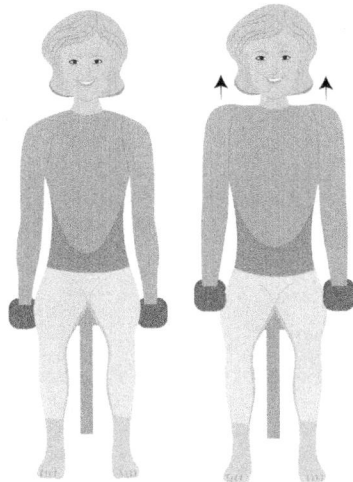

- Begin by sitting on a sturdy chair or bench with your back straight, feet flat on the ground, and knees at a 90-degree angle.
- Hold a dumbbell in each hand by your sides, palms facing your body.
- Keep your arms fully extended and your shoulders relaxed.
- Engage your core muscles by pulling your belly button toward your spine.
- Start the exercise by lifting both shoulders straight up toward your ears while exhaling.
- Keep your arms extended and your back straight.
- Squeeze your shoulder blades together at the top of the shrug.
- Hold the raised position for a moment, feeling the contraction in the muscles between your shoulders and neck.
- Lower your shoulders back down to the starting position while inhaling.
- Maintain a controlled pace throughout the exercise.
- Repeat the exercise 8 to 12 times.
- Perform 2 to 5 sets.

To make it easier, start with lighter dumbbells to reduce the resistance.

You could also perform the exercise one shoulder at a time if using both feels too challenging.

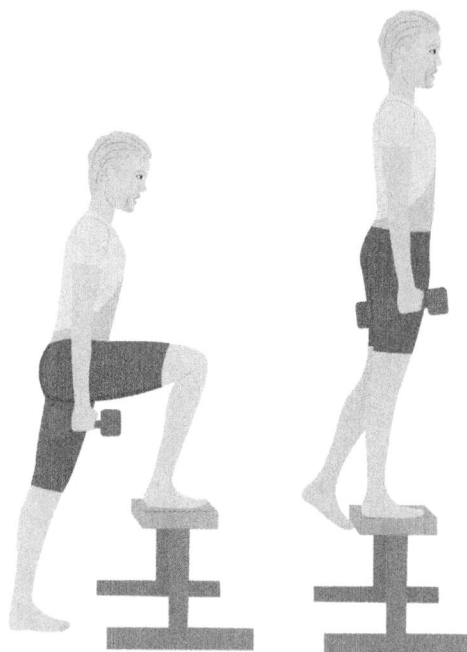

- Begin by standing in front of a sturdy bench or step platform with a dumbbell in each hand.
- Position your feet hip-width apart.
- Keep your back straight, shoulders relaxed, and core engaged.
- Hold the dumbbells by your sides with your palms facing your thighs.
- Place your right foot on the bench or step platform.
- Start the exercise by pressing through your right heel and lifting your body up onto the step while exhaling.
- Fully extend your right leg as you step onto the bench, and place your left foot beside your right foot.
- Ensure that your entire foot is securely on the bench.
- Hold the raised position for a moment, maintaining balance and stability.
- Lower your left foot back down to the ground while inhaling.
- Step down with your right foot, returning to the starting position.
- Repeat the exercise, this time leading with your left foot.
- Alternate between the right and left foot 8 to 15 times.
- Perform 2 to 4 sets.

To make it easier, use a lower bench or step platform to reduce the height of the step-up.

You could also perform the exercise without dumbbells if needed for added stability.

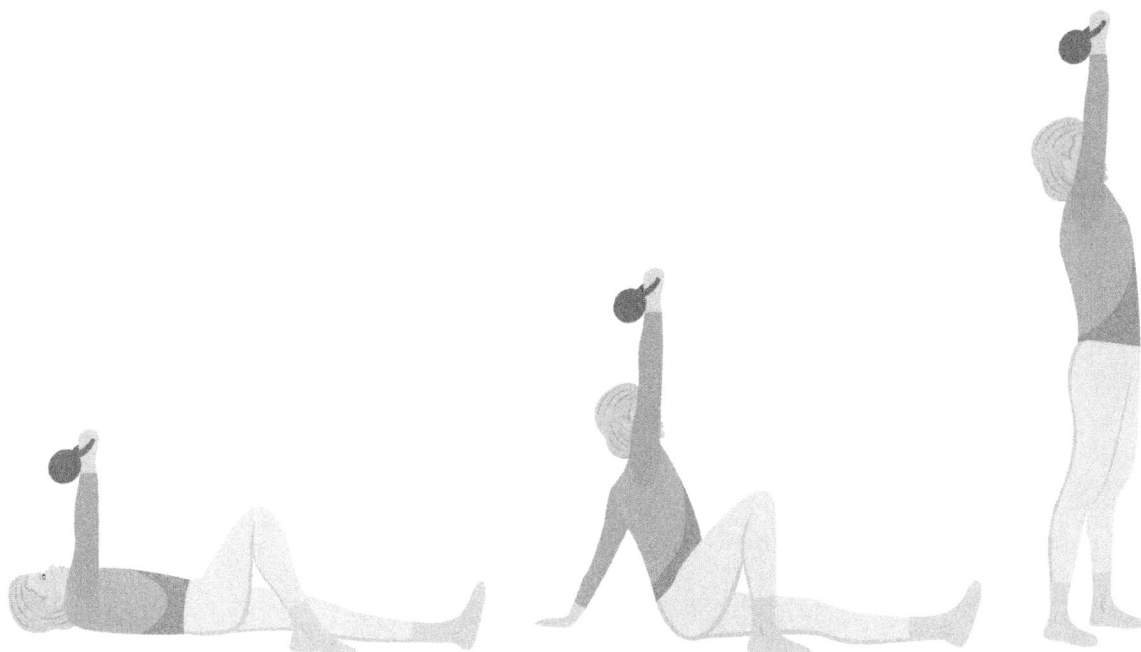

- Begin by lying on your back on a comfortable surface, like a yoga mat.
- Use a light weight or no weight at all to start.
- Roll to your side and use your elbow to prop yourself up.
- Transition from your elbow to your hand to lift your upper body off the ground.
- Raise your hips off the ground by extending your legs and supporting your weight on one knee.
- Continue to push through your hand and raise your torso into a kneeling position.
- Stand up from the kneeling position.
- Reverse the steps to return to the starting position, carefully lowering yourself back to the ground.
- Repeat 8 to 10 times.
- Perform 2 to 3 sets.

To make this easier, use a cushion or soft surface for comfort during the exercise.

You could also reduce the range of motion if necessary, such as not fully extending the arm or not standing fully upright.

Cool Down Stretches

Cool down stretches are vital to do immediately after you've completed your workout. They are beneficial as they help reduce muscle soreness, improve flexibility, and relax the mind.

QUADRICEPS STRETCH | *DIFFICULTY–BEGINNER*

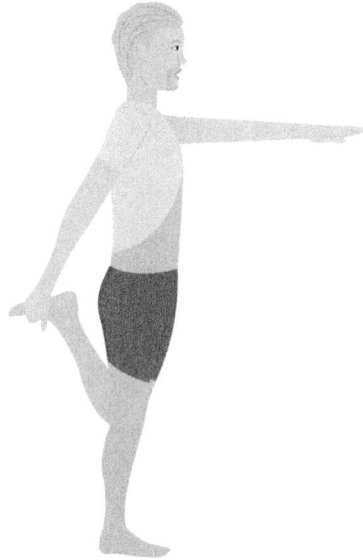

- Stand upright with your feet hip-width apart.
- Shift your weight onto your left leg.
- Bend your right knee, bringing your heel toward your buttocks.
- Reach back with your right hand and grab your right ankle or foot.
- Gently pull your heel closer to your buttocks while keeping your knees together.
- Hold the stretch for 15 to 30 seconds, feeling a mild tension in the front of your thigh.

Release the stretch and switch to the other leg.

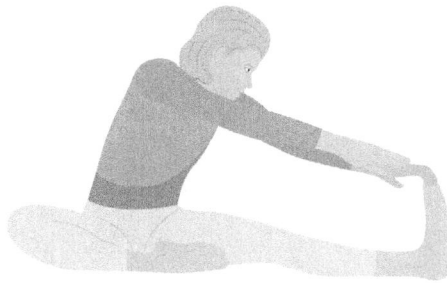

- Sit on the floor with your legs extended straight in front of you.
- Keep your back straight and your toes pointing upward.
- Inhale as you reach both arms overhead.
- Exhale as you hinge at your hips and reach forward toward your toes.
- Keep your back straight, and avoid rounding your spine.
- Hold the stretch for 15 to 30 seconds while breathing deeply.
- Slowly sit back up, releasing the stretch.

Remember to perform each stretch gently and smoothly, without bouncing or forcing your body into uncomfortable positions. Stretch to the point of tension, but not pain, and hold each stretch for an adequate duration to allow your muscles to relax and elongate.

Chapter 4

4-WEEK STRENGTH TRAINING PROGRAM

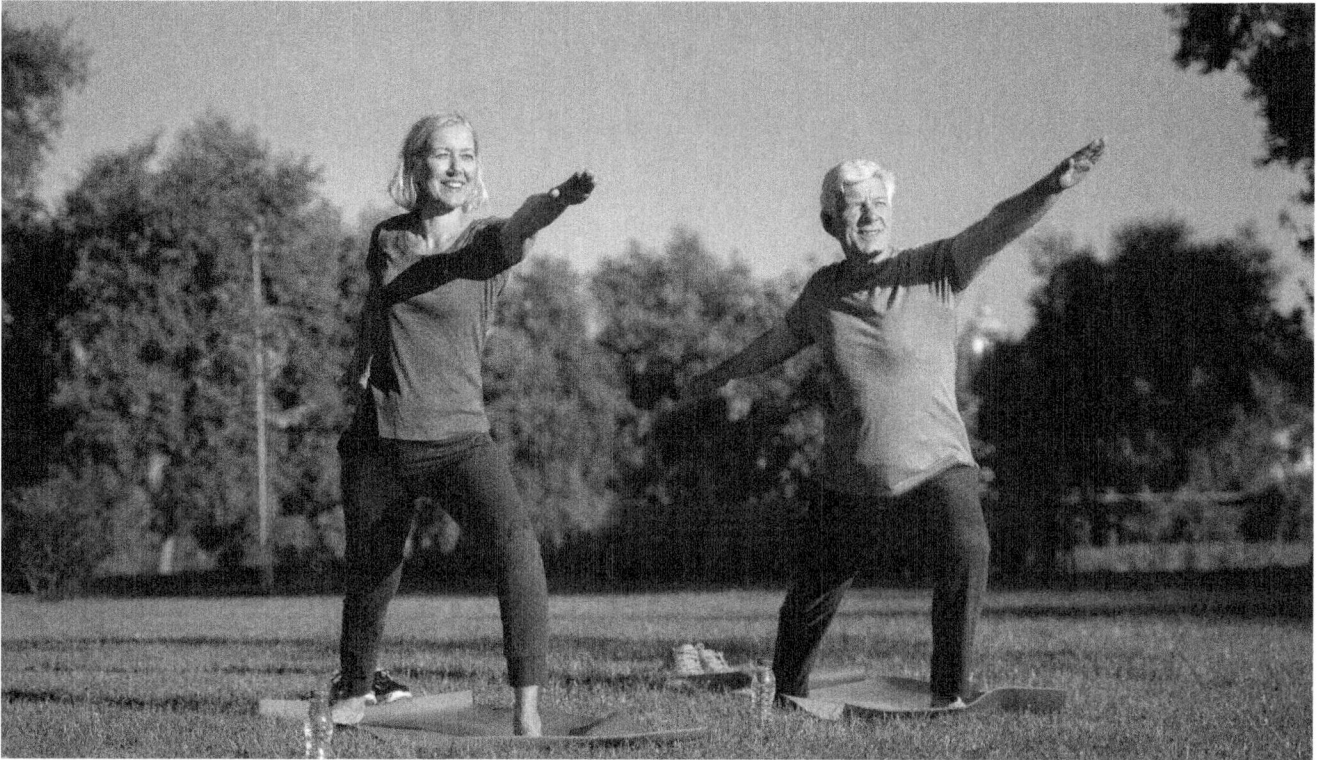

Most of the time we assume that by having the knowledge we will automatically get started, continue with the journey, and succeed in incorporating a certain something into our daily habits. This however is not true. Just because we have the information and knowledge does not mean that we are going to put it to use.

You have the knowledge; a treasure trove of 50 strength training exercises, along with warm-ups, cool-downs, and some beneficial stretching exercises all designed to suit your needs. Now it's time to see how you can slit in a few minutes of exercise into your daily routines. Let's look at a 4-week plan that's specifically designed to help you get stronger each day. The exercises are laid out simply with references to the page where you find the exercise steps and illustrations, as well as how you need to perform them.

Let's get started.

WEEK 1: KICKING OFF YOUR STRENGTH JOURNEY

Day 1

Exercise	Page	Repetitions
Bodyweight Squats	34	Perform 8 to 15 reps and 2 to 4 sets
Dumbbell Lunges	45	Perform 10 to 15 reps and 2 to 5 sets
Seated Dumbbell Shoulder Press	47	Perform 10 to 15 reps and 2 to 3 sets
Standing Leg Calf Raises	39	Perform 8 to 15 reps and 2 to 5 sets
Plank	36	Maintain position for 15-30 seconds Perform 3-5 sets

Day 2

Exercise	Page	Repetitions
Superman	77	Perform 6 to 13 reps and 2 to 5 sets
Hanging Lat Stretch	79	Maintain stretch for 15 to 30 seconds Perform 2 to 3 sets
Seated Russian Twists	67	Perform 10 to 15 reps and 2 to 4 sets
Dumbbell Side Raises	65	Perform 8 to 10 reps and 2 to 5 sets
Chest Press	60	Perform 8 to 15 reps and 2 to 5 sets

Day 3

Exercise	Page	Repetitions
Wall Sit	55	Maintain position for 20 to 30 seconds Perform 2 to 5 sets
Calf Stretches	58	Perform 10 to 15 reps and 2 to 5 sets
Resistance Band Chest Press	50	Perform 8 to 15 reps and 2 to 5 sets
Resistance Band Leg Abduction	46	Perform 10 to 15 reps and 2 to 5 sets
Seated Rows	49	Perform 8 to 15 reps and 2 to 5 sets

Day 4		
Bodyweight Squats	34	Perform 8 to 15 reps and 2 to 4 sets
Knee Extensions With Resistance Band	42	Perform 8 to 15 reps and 3 to 5 sets
Seated Dumbbell Shoulder Press	47	Perform 10 to 15 reps and 2 to 5 sets
Bent Knee DeadLifts	48	Perform 10 to 12 reps and 2 to 5 sets
Lying Leg Curls	54	Perform 8 to 15 reps and 2 to 5 sets
Day 5		
Glute Bridge	63	Perform 8 to 10 reps and 2 to 5 sets
Seated Leg Raises	33	Perform 8 to 15 reps and 2 to 4 sets
Bent Over Dumbbell Rows	34	Perform 8 to 10 reps and 2 to 5 sets
Standing Dumbbell Shoulder Press	43	Perform 8 to 15 reps and 3 to 5 sets
Dumbbell Lunges	45	Perform 10 to 15 reps and 2 to 5 sets
Day 6		
Rest		

WEEK 2: BUILDING STRENGTH AND STABILITY

Day 7

Exercise	Page	Repetitions
Jumping Jacks	31	Perform 20 jumps
Wall Push-ups	35	Perform 8 to 15 reps and 2 to 4 sets
Turkish Get-Up	85	Perform 8 to 10 reps and 2 to 5 sets
Dumbbell Tricep Kickbacks	73	Perform 8 to 10 reps and 2 to 5 sets
Forearm Stretch	75	Maintain position for 20 to 30 seconds; 2 to 3 sets

Day 8

Exercise	Page	Repetitions
Bent Knee DeadLifts	48	Perform 10 to 12 reps and 2 to 5 sets
Resistance Band Leg Curls	66	Perform 8 to 10 reps and 2 to 5 sets
Side Twists	57	Perform 8 to 15 reps and 2 to 5 sets
Standing Leg Calf Raises	39	Perform 8 to 15 reps and 2 to 5 sets
Leg Swings	33	Swing each leg 8 to 15 times. Perform 2 to 3 sets.

Day 9

Exercise	Page	Repetitions
Standing Dumbbell Shoulder Press	43	Perform 8 to 10 reps and 2 to 5 sets
Side Leg Raises	64	Perform 8 to 10 reps and 2 to 5 sets
Resistance Band Bicep Curl	41	Perform 8 to 15 reps and 2 to 5 sets
Dumbbell Step-Ups	84	Perform 8 to 10 reps and 2 to 5 sets
Push-ups	62	Perform 8 to 10 reps and 2 to 5 sets

Day 10		
Dumbbell Bent-Over Reverse Flyes	69	Perform 8 to 10 reps and 2 to 5 sets
Bent Knee Push-ups	51	Perform 8 to 15 reps and 2 to 5 sets
Dumbbell Tricep Kickbacks	73	Perform 8 to 12 reps and 2 to 5 sets
Resistance Band Lat Pulldowns	61	Perform 8 to 10 reps and 2 to 5 sets
Standing Dumbbell Shoulder Press	43	Perform 8 to 10 reps and 2 to 5 sets
Day 11		
Chair Dips	59	Perform 8 to 15 reps and 2 to 5 sets
Resistance Band Bicep Curl	41	Perform 8 to 15 reps and 2 to 5 sets
Turkish Get-Up	85	Perform 8 to 10 reps and 2 to 5 sets
Resistance Band Leg Abduction	46	Perform 10 to 15 reps and 2 to 5 sets
Dumbbell Step-Ups	84	Perform 8 to 10 reps and 2 to 5 sets
Day 12		
Rest		

WEEK 3: PUMPING IT UP

Day 13

Stretch	Page	Repetitions
Leg Swings	33	Swing each leg 8 to 15 times. Perform 2 to 3 sets.
Seated Dumbbell Shrugs	83	Perform 8 to 10 reps and 2 to 5 sets
Resistance Band Leg Curls	66	Perform 8 to 10 reps and 2 to 5 sets
Resistance Band Tricep Stretch	53	Perform 8 to 15 reps and 2 to 5 sets
Push-ups	62	Perform 8 to 10 reps and 2 to 5 sets

Day 14

	Page	Repetitions
Seated Dumbbell Shoulder Press	47	Perform 10 to 15 reps and 2 to 5 sets
Dumbbell Side Raises	65	Perform 8 to 10 reps and 2 to 5 sets
Standing Leg Calf Raises	39	Perform 8 to 15 reps and 2 to 5 sets
Bent Knee Push ups	51	Perform 8 to 15 reps and 2 to 5 sets
Forearm Stretch	75	Maintain position for 20 to 30 seconds Perform 2 to 3 sets

Day 15

	Page	Repetitions
Seated Dumbbell Shoulder Press	47	Perform 10 to 15 reps and 2 to 5 sets
Dumbbell Side Raises	65	Perform 8 to 10 reps and 2 to 5 sets
Standing Leg Calf Raises	39	Perform 8 to 15 reps and 2 to 5 sets
Bent Knee Push ups	51	Perform 8 to 15 reps and 2 to 5 sets
Forearm Stretch	75	Maintain position for 20 to 30 seconds Perform 2 to 3 sets

Day 16

Exercise	Page	Instructions
Lying Hamstring Curls With Weights	74	Perform 12 to 15 reps and 4 to 5 sets
Seated Dumbbell Shrugs	83	Perform 8 to 10 reps and 2 to 5 sets
Wall Angels	40	Perform 10 to 15 reps and 4 to 8 sets
Dumbbell Tricep Kickbacks	73	Perform 8 to 10 reps and 2 to 5 sets
Hanging Lat Stretch	79	Maintain stretch for 15 to 30 seconds Perform 2 to 3 sets

Day 17

Exercise	Page	Instructions
Seated Dumbbell Shrugs	83	Perform 8 to 10 reps and 2 to 5 sets
Bent-Over Dumbbell Rows	38	Perform 8 to 10 reps and 2 to 5 sets
Side Twists	57	Perform 8 to 15 reps and 2 to 5 sets
Dumbbell Bent-Over Reverse Flyes	69	Perform 8 to 10 reps and 2 to 5 sets
Forearm Stretch	75	Maintain position for 20 to 30 seconds Perform 2 to 3 sets

Day 18

Rest

WEEK 4: STRONG AND FLEXIBLE

Day 19

Asana/Stretch	Page	Repetitions
Chair Dips	59	Perform 8 to 15 reps and 2 to 5 sets
Side Twists	57	Perform 8 to 15 reps and 2 to 5 sets
Push-ups	62	Perform 8 to 10 reps and 2 to 5 sets
Resistance Band Bicep Curl	41	Perform 8 to 15 reps and 2 to 5 sets
Calf Stretches	58	Perform 10 to 15 reps and 2 to 5 sets

Day 20

Asana/Stretch	Page	Repetitions
Resistance Band Lat Pulldowns	61	Perform 8 to 10 reps and 2 to 5 sets
Seated Russian Twists	67	Perform 10 to 15 reps and 2 to 5 sets
Resistance Band Leg Curls	66	Perform 8 to 10 reps and 2 to 5 sets
Bent-Over Dumbbell Rows	38	Perform 8 to 10 reps and 2 to 5 sets
Turkish Get-Up	85	Perform 8 to 10 reps and 2 to 5 sets

Day 21

Asana/Stretch	Page	Repetitions
Lying Leg Curls	54	Perform 8 to 15 reps and 2 to 5 sets
Side Bends	80	Perform 6 to 15 reps and 2 to 5 sets
Dumbbell Step-Ups	84	Perform 8 to 10 reps and 2 to 5 sets
Side Twists	57	Perform 8 to 15 reps and 2 to 5 sets
Bent Knee push ups	51	Perform 8 to 15 reps and 2 to 5 sets

Day 22		
Dumbbell Bent-Over Reverse Flyes	69	Perform 8 to 10 reps and 2 to 5 sets
Seated Lateral Raises	70	Perform 8 to 10 reps and 2 to 5 sets
Dumbbell Tricep Kickbacks	73	Perform 8 to 12 reps and 2 to 5 sets
Resistance Band Lat Pulldowns	61	Perform 8 to 10 reps and 2 to 5 sets
Chair Dips	59	Perform 8 to 15 reps and 2 to 5 sets
Day 23		
Toe Touches	78	Perform 12 to 15 reps and 3 to 5 sets
Bodyweight Squats	34	Perform 8 to 15 reps and 2 to 4 sets
Lying Hamstring Curls With Weights	74	Perform 12 to 15 reps and 4 to 5 sets
Plank	36	Maintain position for 20 to 30 seconds Perform 2 to 3 sets
Turkish Get-Up	85	Perform 8 to 10 reps and 2 to 5 sets
Day 24		
Rest		

STRETCH AND RECOVERY WEEK

Day 25

Stretch	Page	Repetitions
Calf Stretches	58	Perform 10 to 15 reps and 2 to 5 sets
Wall Angels	40	Perform 10 to 15 reps and 4 to 8 sets
Resistance Band Hip Abduction	68	Perform 8 to 10 reps and 2 to 5 sets
Bridge With Leg Lifts	71	Perform 8 to 10 reps and 2 to 5 sets
Quadriceps Stretch	86	Hold for 15 seconds. Perform 3 reps and 2 sets on each leg.

Day 26

Calf Stretches	58	Perform 10 to 15 reps and 2 to 5 sets
Toe Touches	78	Perform 10 to 15 repetitions and 2 to 3 sets
Resistance Band Tricep Stretch	53	Perform 8 to 15 reps and 2 to 5 sets
Bridge With Leg Lifts	71	Perform 8 to 10 reps and 2 to 5 sets
Leg Swings	82	Swing each leg 8 to 15 times. Perform 2 to 3 sets.

Day 27

Glute Bridge	63	Perform 8 to 10 reps and 2 to 5 sets
Lying Leg Raises	52	Perform 8 to 15 reps and 2 to 5 sets
Hip Circles	81	Move for 15 to 30 seconds. Perform 2 to 3 sets.
Quadriceps Stretch	86	Hold the position for 15 seconds. Perform 3 reps and 2 sets on each leg.
Side Twists	57	Perform 8 to 15 reps and 2 to 5 sets

Day 28		
Hanging Lat Stretch	79	Maintain stretch for 15 to 30 seconds Perform 2 to 3 sets
Arm Swings	76	Swing for 30 to 60 seconds. Perform 2-3 sets
Side Bends	80	Perform 6 to 15 reps and 2 to 5 sets
Side Twists	57	Perform 8 to 15 reps and 2 to 5 sets
Wall Angels	40	Perform 10 to 15 reps and 4 to 8 sets
Day 29		
Hip Circles	81	Move for 15 to 30 seconds. Perform 2 to 3 sets.
Arm Swings	76	Swing for 30 to 60 seconds. Perform 2-3 sets
Superman	77	Perform 6 to 12 repetitions and 2 to 3 sets
Leg Swings	82	Swing each leg 8 to 15 times. Perform 2 to 3 sets.
Forearm Stretch	75	Maintain position for 20 to 30 seconds Perform 2 to 3 sets
Day 30		
Rest		

Monitoring Progress, Celebrating Achievements, and Empowering You

As we come closer to the end, it's vital that you make sure you have all the tools and knowledge you need to not only stay motivated but also monitor your progress effectively. Let's dive into how you can track your journey and keep pushing your boundaries.

It's important to monitor your progress and celebrate your achievements. Seeing your progress is not just motivating; it's also a powerful way to stay on track. For this reason, it's time for that special gift for you.

The "ForeverFit Progress Journal"

As part of our commitment to your success, you deserve the "ForeverFit Progress Journal." This printable journal is designed to help you:

- Track your workouts and exercises.
- Record your sets, reps, and weights.
- Monitor changes in your strength and endurance.
- Celebrate your achievements, no matter how small.
- Set new goals and milestones.

To access your "ForeverFit Progress Journal," simply scan the QR code provided below, and it will take you to the download page. Print it out, and let it be your constant companion on your fitness journey. It's not just a journal; it's your personal record of strength and achievement.

Tips for Increasing Strength and Resistance

Now, let's talk about how you can take your strength training to the next level by incorporating home equipment and tools. While our workouts are designed to be accessible without any special equipment, adding a few tools to your arsenal can provide additional resistance and variety to your routine.

Resistance Bands

Resistance bands are versatile and affordable. They come in various resistance levels, allowing you to start at a comfortable level and gradually increase the challenge. You can use them for exercises like bicep curls, leg lifts, or lateral raises. The bands are gentle on joints, making them an excellent choice.

Dumbbells

Dumbbells are a classic choice for strength training. They come in different weights, and you can easily adjust the intensity of your exercises by choosing the right pair. Dumbbells can be used for exercises such as squats, lunges, and overhead presses. They offer stability and control, helping you maintain proper form.

Chair Exercises

Don't underestimate the power of a sturdy chair. It can be a valuable piece of equipment for seated leg lifts, step-ups, or tricep dips. A chair provides stability and support while allowing you to work multiple muscle groups.

Water Bottles or Cans

No dumbbells? No problem! Grab two water bottles or cans of equal weight, and you've got makeshift weights for exercises like lateral raises or front raises. These household items are readily available and can be used to add resistance to your workouts.

Remember, whether you choose to incorporate equipment or stick with bodyweight exercises, the key is to challenge yourself safely and progressively. With consistency, dedication, and the right tools, you'll continue to strengthen your body and achieve your fitness goals.

As you embark on your fitness journey armed with the "ForeverFit Progress Journal" and new equipment ideas, keep in mind that you have the power to shape your strength and health in your golden years. Your commitment, effort, and resilience will pay off in improved vitality, mobility, and an overall enhanced quality of life.

Stay strong, stay motivated, and embrace the strength that's within you. Your golden years are meant to shine brightly, and with the right mindset and the tools at your disposal, you're well on your way to a healthier, stronger, and more vibrant you.

Chapter 5

HOW TO BECOME MOTIVATED AND BUILD SELF-DISCIPLINE

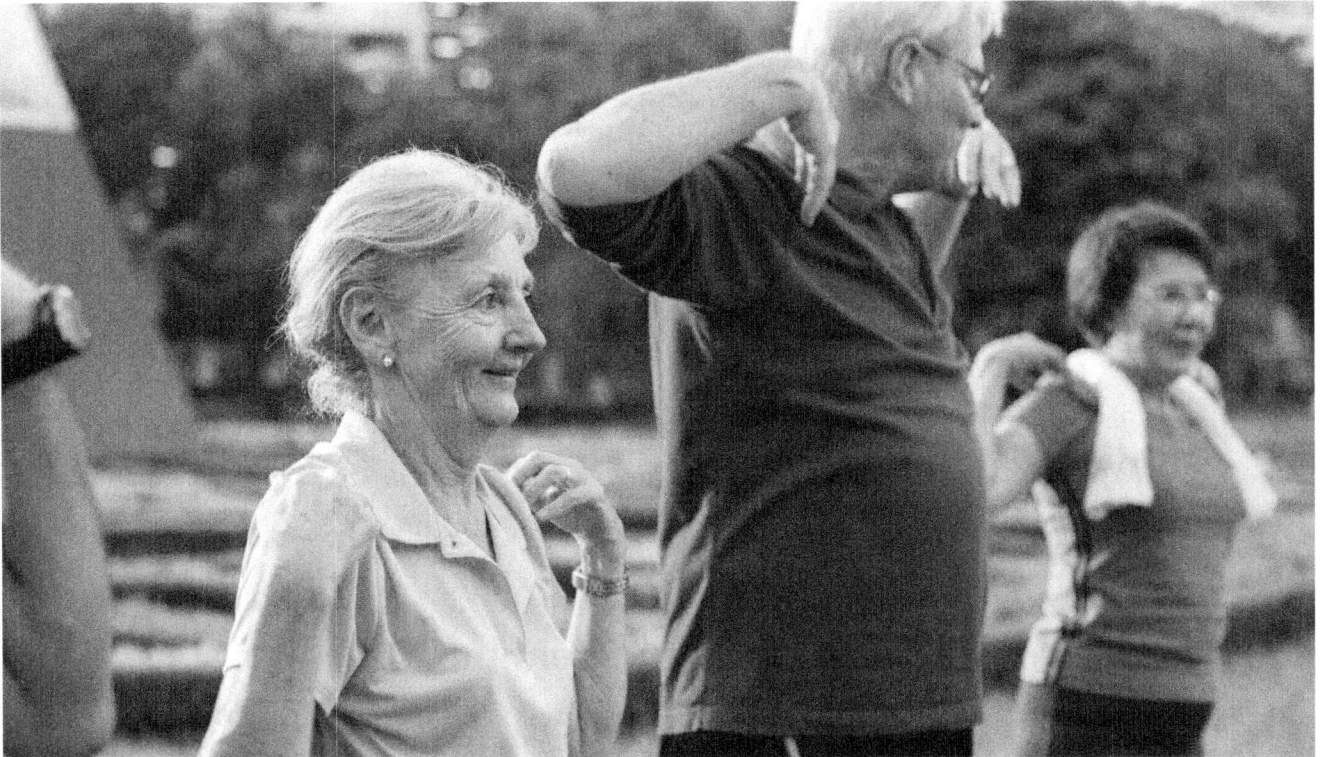

In this chapter, we will delve into the essential elements of motivation and self-discipline that can empower you in your fitness journey. By the end of this chapter, you will have a clear understanding of how to cultivate the mindset and habits necessary for success.

Understanding the Power of a Growth Mindset

First things first, what exactly is this "growth mindset" we keep talking about? Well, a growth mindset is all about believing that your abilities and intelligence can improve over time with effort and practice. It's the opposite of a "fixed mindset," which believes that your talents and intelligence are stuck and cannot improve.

Now, you might wonder, why does this matter for me? Well, here's the thing: As we age, it's easy to fall into the trap of thinking, "I'm too old to change" or "I can't do that anymore." However, a growth mindset challenges these beliefs. It's like saying, "I can learn and improve at any age."

Imagine a senior who thinks, "I can't lift weights; I'm too old." That's a fixed mindset.

On the other hand, a senior with a growth mindset says, "I may not be able to lift much now, but with practice, I can get stronger."

How a Growth Mindset Can Benefit Seniors in Their Fitness Journey

Let's bring this to life with some examples:

Challenging the "I Can't" mentality with a growth mindset, you are more likely to take on new exercises or fitness routines, even if they seem challenging at first. You will see these challenges as opportunities for growth, not as roadblocks.

Picture a senior who faces a setback like a minor injury. A growth mindset helps them view it as a temporary obstacle, not a permanent setback. They'll focus on rehab, recovery, and getting back on track.

Those with a growth mindset are curious learners. They're open to trying different exercises, techniques, or nutrition plans because they believe they can learn and adapt.

In a nutshell, a growth mindset is like opening the door to endless possibilities. It's about believing that, no matter your age, you can always learn, improve, and achieve your fitness goals. So, embrace that growth mindset, and let it be your guiding star on your fitness journey.

The Relationship Between Diet and Strength

Now, let's talk about something that's the backbone of your fitness journey–your diet! Nutrition is like the fuel that powers your body, and for seniors, it plays a crucial role in health and strength.

The Importance of Nutrition

Imagine your body as a finely-tuned machine, and food is the fuel that keeps it running smoothly. Nutrition is especially vital for seniors because it directly impacts their health and fitness. Here's why:

Energy Boost

The right nutrients provide you with the energy you need to stay active and engaged in your fitness routine.

Muscle Maintenance

As we age, we naturally lose muscle mass. Proper nutrition helps seniors maintain muscle strength, which is crucial for balance, mobility, and overall strength.

Bone Health

Certain nutrients, like calcium and vitamin D, are essential for strong bones. This is particularly important for the prevention of fractures and osteoporosis.

How a Balanced Diet Contributes to Strength and Vitality

A balanced diet is like a superhero's toolkit. It includes a variety of foods that provide a range of essential nutrients. Here's how it contributes to strength and vitality:

Proteins for Muscle

Protein-rich foods, like lean meats, fish, beans, and nuts, help build and repair muscle. They also keep you feeling full and satisfied.

Vitamins and Minerals

Fruits and vegetables are packed with vitamins and minerals that support overall health. For example, vitamin C helps with tissue repair, while potassium aids in muscle function.

The Value of Hydration

Don't forget about water! Staying hydrated is essential for maintaining energy levels, lubricating joints, and regulating body temperature.

Practical Tips on Senior-Specific Dietary Choices

Protein-Packed Meals

Include a source of lean protein in each meal, such as chicken, fish, tofu, or legumes. This supports muscle strength and helps with your recovery after workouts.

Fiber for Digestion

Fiber-rich foods like whole grains, fruits, and vegetables are essential for digestive health. They also keep you feeling full and satisfied.

Calcium and Vitamin D

Incorporate dairy products, fortified cereals, or supplements if needed to ensure you're getting enough calcium and vitamin D for strong bones.

Stay Hydrated

Make it a habit to drink water throughout the day, especially before, during, and after exercise. Dehydration can lead to muscle cramps and fatigue.

Limit Sugary and Processed Foods

Minimize foods and drinks high in added sugars and processed ingredients. These can contribute to weight gain and negatively impact your overall health.

Remember, your diet is a key player in your fitness journey. By making mindful choices and embracing a balanced diet, you're not just fueling your body; you're also setting the stage for strength, vitality, and an active lifestyle.

Cheers to healthy eating.

Setting and Achieving Goals

Setting and achieving fitness goals can be a game-changer on your journey to staying active and healthy. Here's why it matters and how to make it work for you:

The Significance of Setting Fitness Goals for Motivation

Think of your fitness goals as your guiding stars. They give you a clear direction and purpose. Setting goals:

Boosts Motivation

When you have a goal in mind, whether it's to walk a certain distance or lift a specific weight, it gives you something to strive for. It's like having a finish line in a race that keeps you going.

Provides Focus

Goals help you concentrate your efforts. You're more likely to stick with a workout routine when you know it's getting you closer to your desired outcome.

Setting Realistic and Achievable Fitness Goals

Now, the key to successful goal-setting is to:

Be Realistic

Set goals that are attainable based on your current fitness level. If you've never run before, aiming to complete a marathon next month might not be the best start. Instead, start with smaller, achievable milestones.

Make Them Specific

The more specific your goal, the easier it is to track progress. For example, "I want to be able to do ten push-ups without stopping" is more concrete than "I want to get stronger."

Break It Down

Sometimes, big goals can be overwhelming. Break them into smaller, manageable steps. This way, you can celebrate your progress along the way.

Tracking Progress and Celebrating Achievements

Tracking progress is like keeping score in a game-it shows you how well you're doing and where you can improve.

Keep a Workout Journal

Write down your exercises, sets, reps and any notes about how you felt during the workout. This journal becomes a record of your journey and a source of motivation.

Celebrate Achievements

Don't forget to celebrate your victories, no matter how small. Every step counts! It could be treating yourself to a healthy snack or sharing your success with a friend.

Building Self-Discipline

Self-discipline is like your personal trainer for sticking to your fitness routine. Here's how you can cultivate it:

Set a Routine

Establish a consistent workout schedule. When exercise becomes a habit, it's easier to stick with it.

Find Accountability

Partner up with a friend or join a fitness group. Knowing that someone else is counting on you can be a powerful motivator.

Stay Positive

Focus on the positive aspects of exercise. Instead of thinking, "I have to work out," say, "I get to work out, and it makes me feel great!"

The Benefits of Consistent and Disciplined Fitness Routines

The rewards of self-discipline are worth the effort.

Improved Health

Consistency in exercise can lead to better heart health, increased mobility, and a reduced risk of chronic diseases.

Enhanced Well-Being

Regular physical activity releases endorphins, which boost mood and reduce stress. It's like a natural happiness pill.

Longevity

A disciplined fitness routine can contribute to a longer and more active life, allowing you to enjoy the things you love for longer.

Overcoming Common Challenges

Challenges are a part of any fitness journey, but they can be conquered. Some challenges include

- lack of time.
- injuries or health concerns.
- weather and environment.

Solutions and Coping Strategies for Addressing These Challenges

- Prioritize your health. Even short, frequent workouts can be effective.
- If you have health concerns, consult a healthcare provider or a fitness expert to create a safe and effective workout plan.
- When the weather is uncooperative, consider indoor exercises like dancing, yoga, or home workouts.

Keep pushing forward, and remember, challenges are just opportunities in disguise!

Maintaining Motivation Over Time

So, you've set goals, built self-discipline, and conquered challenges. Now, the final piece of the puzzle is maintaining that motivation for the long haul.

Strategies for Sustaining Motivation in the Long Term

Variety is the Spice of Life

Keep your workouts fresh by trying different activities. It could be swimming, hiking, or even dancing. New experiences can reignite your passion for fitness.

Find Your "Why"

Revisit your reasons for embarking on this fitness journey. Your "why" is your anchor during moments when motivation wanes.

Set New Goals

As you achieve your initial goals, set new ones to keep the excitement alive. This keeps you focused and continually progressing.

The Importance of Adapting and Evolving Your Fitness Routine

Remember, your body changes over time, so your fitness routine should too. You must:

Listen to Your Body

Pay attention to how your body responds to exercise. Adjust your routine if something doesn't feel right or if you want to challenge yourself more.

Incorporate Variety

Include a mix of cardio, strength training, flexibility, and balance exercises. This holistic approach benefits your overall well-being.

Stay Informed

Stay up-to-date with the latest fitness trends and information. Learning something new can reignite your enthusiasm.

Support Networks for You to Stay Motivated

Don't go it alone! There's strength in numbers.

- Join a group: Find a local fitness group or class where you can meet like-minded individuals. The camaraderie and shared goals can be incredibly motivating.
- Online communities: Explore online forums or social media groups dedicated to senior fitness. You can share your experiences, seek advice, and find inspiration.
- Family and friends: Share your fitness journey with loved ones. They can provide encouragement and even join you in your workouts.

We've covered a lot in this chapter, and now you know that you must believe in your ability to learn and improve, no matter your age. A balanced diet fuels your strength and vitality. Set clear, achievable goals for motivation. Cultivate discipline to stay committed to your fitness routine. Identify and conquer common obstacles. Keep the fire burning for the long term.

Now, it's over to you. Apply these principles, take small steps every day, and embrace a fit and disciplined lifestyle. Remember, your journey is unique, and every effort counts. Stay motivated, stay strong, and enjoy the rewards of a healthier, happier you!

CONCLUSION

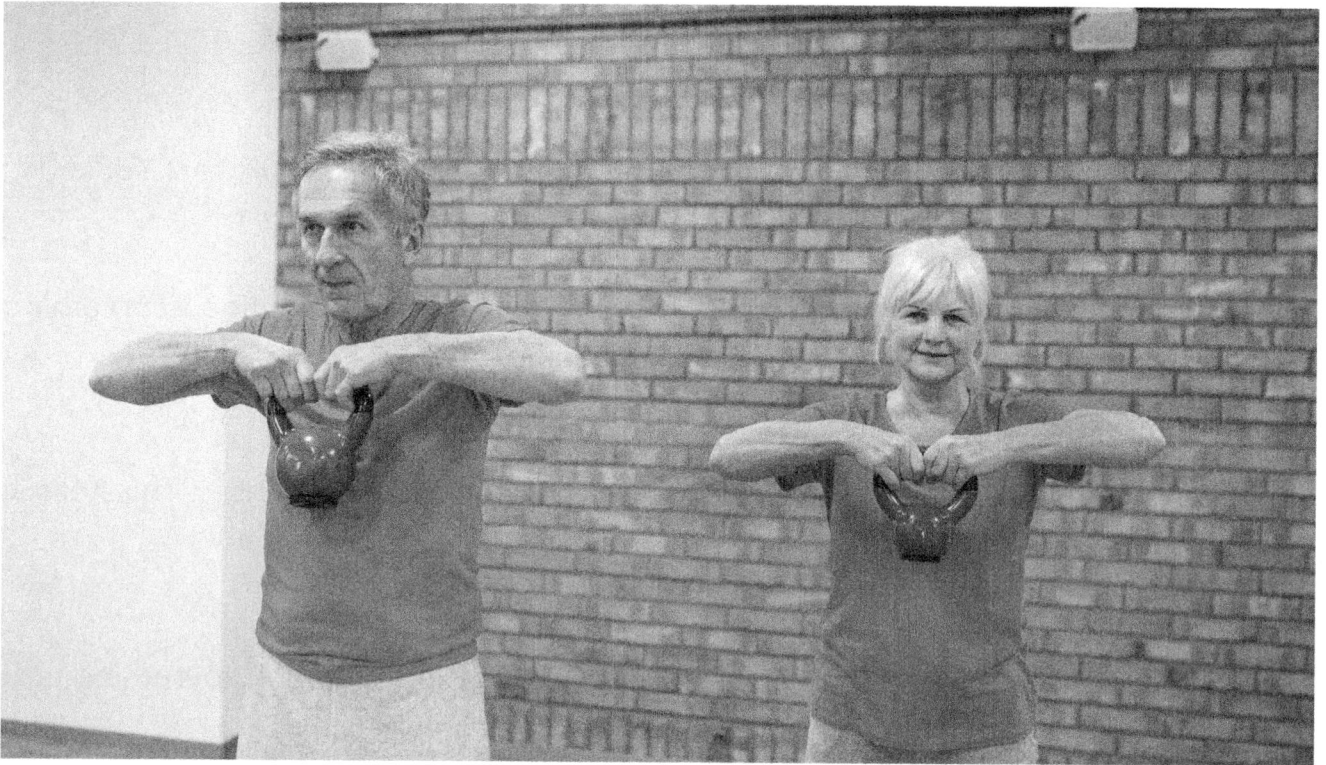

As we reach the end of our journey through "5-Minute Strength Training Workouts for Seniors," it's time to reflect on the wealth of knowledge and guidance that this book has to offer. Throughout these chapters, we've explored the path to strength, health, and vitality in the golden years. Let's summarize the key takeaways and leave you with some final words of encouragement.

This book has been a companion on your quest for strength and health. In Chapter 1, we discussed the importance of being strong and healthy in your golden years. We emphasized how incorporating strength workouts can benefit your overall health and metabolism. We addressed issues like immobility, muscle fatigue, and weakness, providing you with strategies to overcome these challenges. We also debunked myths about strength training as we age, paving the way for a new understanding of what's possible.

In Chapter 2, we introduced you to the world of strength and resistance training, showcasing how it can be gentle, low-impact, and accessible to everyone. We emphasized the immense benefits seniors can reap by becoming strong and healthy.

Chapter 3 was a treasure trove of 50 strength and resistance training exercises, each presented with clear illustrations and instructions, catering to different difficulty levels. These exercises provide you with a toolbox to craft your personalized fitness routine.

In Chapter 4, we guided you through a weekly breakdown of the 50 exercises from Chapter 3. We gave each week a name representing its purpose, ensuring you understood that you should work within your limitations while striving for new goals. We emphasized the importance of monitoring progress and celebrating achievements, offering you the "ForeverFit Progress Journal" as a tool to track your success.

Chapter 5 introduced the concept of a growth mindset, showing why it's crucial for seniors. We connected the dots between a good diet and strength training, underscoring the synergy between proper nutrition and physical strength. We discussed how you can make smart workout choices to maximize your fitness journey.

Throughout this book, one resounding message has been clear: With the right mindset and persistence, you can achieve whatever strength goals you set. Your age is not a barrier; it's a badge of experience and wisdom. Embracing strength and health in your golden years is not just about looking better; it's about feeling better, moving better, and living better.

As you continue your journey towards greater strength and health, here are some additional tips to consider:

- If you wish to enhance your workouts, consider investing in some simple home equipment like resistance bands, dumbbells, or stability balls. These tools can add variety and resistance to your exercises.
- Consistency is key to reaping the benefits of strength training. Stick to your routine and remember that progress may be gradual, but it's worth it.
- Don't forget the importance of rest and recovery days. Your body needs time to heal and grow stronger between workouts.
- Keep learning and staying informed about the latest trends and research in senior fitness. Knowledge is a powerful tool on your journey.

In closing, *5-Minute Strength Training Workouts for Seniors* is not just a book; it's your guide to a healthier, stronger, and more vibrant life. Whether you're a senior looking to maintain your strength or someone who cares about the well-being of a senior in your life, the principles and exercises within these pages can make a profound difference.

Remember, it's never too late to start, and every small step you take toward a healthier, stronger you is a victory. Embrace the knowledge and wisdom shared in this book, and let it be your companion on your lifelong journey to health and strength. You've got this, and your golden years can shine even brighter with the power of strength and resilience.

Without your voice we don't exist.
Please, support us and leave a honest review on Amazon

Just scan this QR code with your phone's camera and leave a review

SCAN
ME

Printed in Great Britain
by Amazon

39335975R00064